MW01711514

the **missing cornerstone**

Reasons why couples choose Natural Family Planning in their marriage

S. Joseph Tham, M.D.

Circle Press

Copyright © 2003 Circle Press
Circle Press is a program of Circle Media Inc.
33 Rossotto Dr.
Hamden, CT 06514 USA
1-203-230-0729

All rights reserved. No part of this book may be used or reproduced in any manner whatsoever without permission from the publisher.

Cover design by María Eugenia Saiz
Printed in the United States of America

ISBN 0-9651601-9-X

Library of Congress Control Number: 2003107548

Preface

When the contraceptive pill was introduced in about 1960 it was promoted internationally with intensive propaganda, as a result of which a massive commercial enterprise developed. Gradually disillusionment occurred because of the complications produced by the medication, some resulting from the synthetic estrogen component and others related to the synthetic progestogen. The blood-clotting occurred in veins and sometimes caused fatal pulmonary embolism, but obstruction also occurred in major arteries in the heart, the brain or in the limbs. Efforts were made to prevent the blood clotting by lowering the dose of the estrogen which reduced but not eliminate the problem. As well as that a number of pregnancies were occurring in spite of women following the instructions of usage correctly. New formulations were engineered with the marketing of second generation and later third generation pills, and administration was accomplished by subcutaneous implants or injections. The toxicity increased.

It is time to face the truth. The attempt to prevent births by the administration of medication, which obviously involves the suppression or even destruction of elements of a normally functioning, complex and important biological system, will inevitably produce serious complications in at least a proportion of those who are persuaded to adopt such a recommendation. The woman and her husband should decide whether it is wise to ingest drugs which cause a variety of unpleasant symptoms and continue to carry risks of serious complications, or will choose a natural method of regulating fertility which is highly effective for the postponement of pregnancy and is becoming the primary management of a problem of infertility. It also helps the woman to seek early diagnosis and treatment of any gynaecological abnormality that disturbs the cycle, and promotes generosity and deeper love between husband and wife, leading to peace, happiness and security within the marriage. This book will help couples to understand and make good decisions.

JOHN J. BILLINGS, M.D.
Founder and president of the Billings Ovulation Method as recognized by the World Health Organization. Both he and his wife have served on several ad hoc committees for the WHO.

THIS BOOK IS DEDICATED TO

MARY,

QUEEN OF THE FAMILY

Acknowledgments

Many people have generally offered their time and help in order for this work to become a reality. First, I would like extend my sincere gratitude to Archbishop Chaput of Denver who kindly permitted his pastoral letter on Human Life of 1984 to be included in the appendix. I would like to thank especially the couples who contributed their personal testimonies that make up the bulk of this book. Their lives are eloquent examples of dedication and fidelity. I would also like to thank Drs John and Evelyn Billings, Dr Thomas Hilgers, and Dr John Kippley in their support of this work by offering their prudent advice and recommendations. Dr John Billings has been most meticulous in sending me corrections and suggestions, as well as writing a paragraph about this book. Dr John Kippley offered to insert my request for testimonies into the CCL bimonthly newsletter. I would like to thank Fr Gene Livosa who sent me two newspaper articles which have been included. Among those who agreed to read my first draft and offered their opinions and corrections, their help has been invaluable. They are the following: Fr Michael Ryan, LC, Fr Gonzalo Miranda, LC and Fr Thomas Williams, LC, who are the respective school Deans Philosophy, Bioethics and Theology at the *Pontifical Atheneum Regina Apostolorum*; Dr Janet Smith, Professor of Philosophy, University of Dallas; Fr John Comiskey of St Peter's Seminary of London, Ontario; Fr Daniel McCaffrey, STD of the Archdiocese of Oklahoma; Fr Richard Au of the Archdiocese of Vancouver; Sr Marilyn Mangan, CND of *Marguerite Bourgeoys Family Service* in Toronto; Angela and George Fazari; Mr Anthony Hagerty; Mr John Dumont; Dr Lucy Hyndman; Dr Elizabeth Sem and Fr Christopher Bazaanah of Ghana. I would like to thank Mr Jay Good for proofreading the second draft. I would also like to thank the benefactors who contributed in the publication of this work, especially Mr. Michael Weiss. Last but not least, many fellow seminarians in Rome helped out in the scanning and typing of the texts of which I am most grateful.

Other books by Circle Press

Integral Formation of Catholic Priests
Peter on the Shore
Vocation Questions and Answers
Founders
Eucharist through the Centuries
New Woman

Contents

About this book

Once upon a time, in a land far, far away, a King commissioned his best architects to construct a palace for him. The architects gathered to discuss, and to design, this momentous work. They wanted to make sure that it would be the grandest and most beautiful palace ever made in the history of the Kingdom. Among them, however, was an architect who would not participate in the designing, nor the construction, of the palace. Without saying a word, he observed the progress of the building. Some days, he was found alone working on a particular brick, measuring, chiseling and polishing it. Nobody knew what he was up to. They all thought that he was crazy and began calling him "Fool." After years of toil, the great day came when the palace was finished. The architects organized a big celebration and invited the King to come for the opening ceremony. Just before the arrival of the King, however, the architects discovered a grave oversight — the cornerstone was missing! Without this, the palace was in imminent danger of collapse. What a disaster! There was not enough time to make a new cornerstone. It was then that one of the workers exclaimed, "That brick that the Fool was working on all these years, maybe it will fit." They rushed to the Fool's house, found the brick and brought it to the palace. And, lo and behold — it fit perfectly. When the King arrived and learned about it, he summoned for the Fool, but the Fool had long since disappeared.

As one gets older, childhood fables often take on new significance. The workers and architects in the story were oblivious to the fact that their work was about to fall apart. Very often in our lives, we become too comfortable with what goes on around us and we lose sight of what really goes on. When someone comes around trying to warn us of danger, we do not take the warning seriously. Yet, this type of happy-go-lucky attitude can often have disastrous consequences.

Our society can be compared to the palace being constructed in the fable. There are usually different opinions as to the best way to go about its construction. Anyone who has been to a construction site will be familiar with its noisy and dust-filled environment. The noises and movements can distract us, and the dust from all around can cloud our vision. As a result, we may easily miss what is going on — the cornerstone of our society is missing, and like the palace in the fable, our society is on the brink of collapse.

If the family unit is the building block of all human societies, it is not too difficult to see that our society is in serious trouble. The modern family is in crisis. One only needs to look at the statistics to see the dramatic rise of the number of broken marriages, single parent families, teenage pregnancies, child abuse, and abortions in the North American.[1] Each of us, I am sure, has been touched by these realities in some way.

What could be the core of this crisis in the family life? What is the missing cornerstone?[2] In 1968, the Pope Paul VI issued an encyclical letter called *Humanae Vitae* that caused a great deal of uproar both inside and outside the Church. The position of this encyclical is well known; he reaffirmed that contraceptive use is not permissible in marriages although natural means to space births are allowed. However, this is only the more publicized part of the message. Many have not been given the chance to hear the positive vision of the Church on the

[1] American Statistics: Pregnancy of unmarried teenagers doubled in last 20 years to one million per year in 1990, resulting in 406,000 abortions. Abortion rates tripled to 1.6 million in 1990 since 1972. Reported cases of child abuse quadrupled from 1976 to 2.7 million cases in 1990. Teen suicide rate has more than tripled from 1960 to 1990 and is the third leading cause of death among adolescents. The number of divorces increased 200% in the last 30 years to 21 divorces per thousand married women in 1987. Less than 60% of all children are living with both their biological married parents in 1990. Seventeen million children live in single-parent homes in1991. *The Index of Leading Cultural Indicators,* Vol. 1, WILLIAM J. BENNETT, 1993.

[2] Interestingly, some social scientists also attribute the rapid deterioration of the Western societies in the last thirty years-increasing crime rate, decreasing trust, changes in family structure, and the triumph of individualism over community-with the advance of birth control. Such a thesis is noted, for example, by Francis Fukuyama, *The Great Disruption: Human Nature and the Reconstitution of Social Order*, The Free Press, New York, 1999, p. 101-103.

meaning and end of human sexuality. At the time *Humanae Vitae* was published, there were dissension and protests. It remains a controversial issue today. Words like 'contraception' and 'Natural Family Planning' are taboo in many Catholic circles and are rarely heard from the pulpits. Besides, many people today still do not understand why the Church has condemned contraceptive use while allowing Natural Family Planning.[3]

Is the radical message of *Humanae Vitae* so often ridiculed by the media and disregarded by many Catholics a foolish one? Or is this really like the message of the Fool in the fable who foresaw the collapse of family life and the moral fabric of society? Can this be the missing cornerstone of the edifice of society — an unheeded message that can explain the present crisis of the family?

After medical school, when I began to practice medicine, I too was faced with this dilemma. Was the message of the Church a foolish one that is to be ignored, or is it a prophetic message? After much personal struggle and research, I came to the realization that it was the latter. When I began to work with couples who were using Natural Family Planning, I saw how the theory of this message — when put into practice — yields marvelous results. The couples whom I met are different from the others who do not use NFP in their marriage. There is something special in the way these spouses treat one another and there is an indescribable aura of joy and contentment about them. Their marriages appear happy and wholesome.

This face of the practice of NFP is often not heard or talked about in the public realm. In fact, I came across a couple of books which claim that NFP is bad for marriages and that most couples suffer from it. I know that not to be the case and felt the need to collect testimonies

[3] Natural Family Planning is planning to achieve or avoid a pregnancy by the timing of intercourse. By observing and recording certain natural symptoms and bodily changes that occur in a woman's menstrual cycle and using the information as a guide, a couple can learn to identify fertile and infertile phases in the menstrual cycle. If the couple wishes to achieve pregnancy, they can be aware of the best days for this to occur. If the couple wishes to avoid pregnancy, they must abstain form genital contact during the fertile cycle. Natural Family Planning for avoiding pregnancy is also referred to as "periodic abstinence". The World Health Organization definition of periodic abstinence is voluntary avoidance of intercourse during the fertile phase of the menstrual cycle in order to avoid pregnancy.

and stories from users of NFP to show a more accurate picture. This was what prompted me to write this book.

In addition, I felt a need to let the people speak of their experiences in their use of Natural Family Planning in their marriage. People nowadays are not too interested in theories or moral doctrines in the air. They are more impressed by practical witnesses rather than empty preaching. With this in mind, I then sent out questionnaires to couples who would be interested in sharing their experiences. I contacted couples whom I know, friends and colleagues who are involved with NFP, and with the various groups who provide NFP services in the States and Canada. The questionnaire was open-ended and was an invitation for the couples to share their personal stories in a format they feel most comfortable.

The response has been quite generous. The testimonies came in many diverse forms. There were talks, stories, dialogues, conferences, and newspaper clippings. They came from couples using different methods of NFP; some started in the 1950's when not much was known about the subject while others began recently. The couples come from people of all walks of life — lawyers, dentists, doctors, housewives, guards, artists, teachers, and construction workers. Most of them came from Americans, with a few from Canada, England, Latin America and even Africa. The motivations to use the natural methods varied as well. Many began due to reasons of faith, while others opted for it for natural and health reasons. There were also stories from doctors who had to struggle with this issue in their practices.

The names and places in these stories have been changed for the sake of anonymity, but they reveal the lives and convictions of many real, actual couples. These testimonies are collected and edited into the present book with the stories written in the first person. It is important to clarify one point — this book is not meant to be a *survey* on the practice of Natural Family Planning. Rather, it is meant to show that there are many who use it and that the demands of *Humanae Vitae* are not unlivable. Certainly, it would be unrealistic to paint the picture of "a rose garden." But it has been amazing for me to see the human spirit at work in times of difficulties. In many stories, it is inspiring to read about the heroic living out of one's faith and to see the work of grace in so many lives.

In a society where more and more people are centered on immediate self-gratification and materialism, love is often promoted as getting what you desire and being fulfilled. But the Christian message is exactly the opposite. Love is not taking but giving — Christ died on the cross not for his own sake but for the sake of others. "To love is to give so much that it hurts," said Mother Teresa of Calcutta. This paradox of love is seen in those who use Natural Family Planning where love implies self-denial and sacrifice.

Although the ills of the North American family life cannot be solely attributed to the use of artificial contraception, the contraceptive mentality — which feeds into egoism and consumerism — has definitely contributed to it. I believe that the cornerstone that has been missing in the construction of a civilization of love, as found in the message of *Humanae Vitae*, is the true notion of human love and human sexuality.

In the sixties, there was much talk about the Sexual Revolution. For some, this revolution meant abandoning all previous social norms and taboos regarding sex. It was regarded by some as a true champion of freedom. Yet, with the sad state of affairs regarding family life today, one must concede that this so-called revolution has been a failure. Perhaps, the time is ripe for a new Sexual Revolution — which is the revolution of love, of true human love. Let these stories speak for themselves and show you that love is possible!

My story

Everyone has his or her own story to tell. It is only fair that I begin with mine...

The year after my medical internship, I was not sure what I was going to do. I began filling in for family doctors who went on vacation (the technical jargon for this is *locums*) and did some house calls. In this way, I could discover the type of medical practice I eventually would like to set up.

Since I had just graduated from medical school, I was more used to treating very sick patients in the teaching hospitals. Hence, it was a change to see and treat patients with common ailments such as colds, stomach flus, ingrown toenails, and ear infections, etc. However, one facet of this work that I did not quite expect was the number of women who came to me asking for birth control information. Some came to renew their monthly birth control pill (BCP) prescription (in Canada, BCP cannot be purchased without a doctor's prescription). Some came to ask for medical advice regarding the different forms of birth controls. Others came for "morning after pills"[4] after an "unprotected" intercourse. They varied from regular housewives to teenage girls in school uniform. The younger girls usually come with other problems of suspected pregnancies and sexually transmitted diseases. In medical school and internship, we were shown and taught the workings of the various methods of birth control and their respective risks and benefits. However, I felt totally unprepared to deal with these questions which were often not strictly medical but ethical as well.

I clearly remember the case of a sixteen-year-old who came to repeat her prescription of BCP which her family doctor had been giving her for the past two years. She had two abortions already. Am I to refuse her further "medications"? I felt totally unprepared to address this complicated issue.

As a committed and practicing Catholic, I knew that the Church teaches that any form of contraception is always wrong. I had read *Humanae Vitae* a few times but still could not decide. I suppose the medical training makes it very difficult to break with the accepted standards of medical practice. Practically, I knew of no Catholic doctors who did not prescribe the pill. I had my training in two Catholic hospitals in a city and they did not differ much in practice from the rest in this regard except they did not offer abortions.

I was not able to obtain much light from my church either. I approached several priests and they all gave different and sometimes contradictory answers. Most said that it was alright; others said 'no', but could not answer my questions satisfactorily. I remember clearly

[4] Morning after pill is a combination of high dose estrogen and progesterone given post-coitally (after sexual intercourse) to induce supposedly an artificial menstruation in the hope that if conception were to take place, the conceptus would be flushed out or prevented from implantation on the uterine wall. Strictly speaking, it is not a method of contraception but of contra-implantation. Hence, it is an abortifacient.

that one priest said that I would not be sinning by prescribing the pill to my patients because my cooperation with this would be considered only 'material'.[5] He suggested that a Catholic doctor who has problems with his conscience on this issue should specialize and not be in family practice in order to avoid the problem. That was not very helpful and I sought to get to the bottom of this. I started to research this topic, getting books on ethics and moral theology, reading as much as I could, and finding out more about Natural Family Planning (NFP). Similarly, I began to curtail my prescribing of the pill and referrals to sterilization procedures. Yet, I felt very hypocritical in that I was not able to offer any reasonable alternatives to artificial contraception.

Around that time, a couple who were friends of mine were getting married. They told me that they had learned about Natural Family Planning from the Marriage Encounter program at their local church and that they had planned to use it in their marriage. They told me that what they had learned was really scientific and they were happy about using it afterwards. This was the first time that I knew of any young couple who consciously opted for NFP in their marriage. This perked my interest to learn more about NFP. All that I remembered from my medical training on this topic was this one-liner from an Obstetric-Gynecology professor, "Rhythm is unreliable."

I went to see about this program of Natural Family Planning that my friends spoke of so highly. Sr. Marilyn Meagan, CND[6] and Dr Theresa McKenna[7] gave me a one-hour presentation on the workings of mod-

[5] The distinction between formal and material cooperation in sin is that while formal cooperation in sin is always illicit, material cooperation in sin is sometimes licit. Formal cooperation means that the cooperator consents, that is shares the intention of the one who is the principal actor in the evil action. Material cooperation means precisely that the cooperator may not share the intention (his will is not consenting to the evil done by the second party), but his action is a material condition for the other evil action to be accomplished. Depending on the degree of involvement, one's material cooperation is either proximate or remote. In this case, a doctor signing a prescription of contraceptives to a woman should be considered a material cooperation in sin. His signature is a condition of possibility for her to get the prescription filled. Whether she can do that with someone else or not is irrelevant. Would this material collaboration be considered as proximate or remote? As a rule of thumb, proximate material collaboration in another's evil is seldom justifiable. In this case, signing that prescription would be a proximate material cooperation.

[6] Creignton Model Natural Family Planning Practitioner, Supervisor and Educator, and member of the American Academy of Natural Family Planning.

[7] Creighton Model Natural Family Planning Practitioner and Medical Consultant.

ern Natural Family Planning. Dr Theresa is an anesthetist but could not practice her medicine because she refuses to work in any operations involving sterilization procedures. There were no hospitals in town which would accept her conditions. I was suitably impressed with their presentation and even more so with their convictions.

However, my previous training was still so fresh that I found it difficult to break with the "accepted standard of medical practice." Doctors in general stick together in deciding what will be considered true medicine or not. Everything new, be they new treatments, procedures or medicines, has to be proven scientifically with experiments under strict control. Hence, anything that does not fall within this realm of medical science is frowned upon. Those doctors who practice outside these accepted norms are often looked upon as 'quacks'. Being a new graduate, I was all too susceptible to the pressure to conform. Yet, I must now raise this question, "Why is a certain branch of medical science so bent on ignoring categorically the evidence of the scientific value of NFP?" When 'science' is selectively biased against certain scientific truths, I wonder if the spirit of science — which is the spirit to seek the truth — is still present. I think that is the case with NFP where there are many interests at work which are ideologically and economically motivated, rather than scientifically based.[8]

Getting back to my experience, I was becoming more convinced of the Church's teaching, and I had to confront this dilemma head-on. The following fall, I enrolled in an intense one-week course for doctors on Natural Family Planning held at Omaha, Nebraska. There, I met Dr. Thomas Hilgers who is an obstetric-gynecology specialist and founder of the Creighton Model of NFP.[9] He was a true inspiration for me because, as a physician and committed Christian, he showed me how it is possible to combine one's faith coherently with one's profession. There were several other physicians at this course

[8] One can see this in that pharmaceutical companies are sponsoring much medical research where their interests are based on the market economy. Almost all of these international companies manufacture birth-control pills; and it is not in their interest to sponsor research that would potentially damage the sale of their pills.

[9] See the Appendix 1 for the different methods of Natural Family Planning.

and we were able to share our experiences. Apart form learning about the medical aspects of NFP and its application. We also learned a bit about the history, philosophy, and moral theology surrounding the issues of contraception, sterilization, abortion and NFP.

During this week, I confessed for the first time the sin of prescribing contraception to a priest and decided once and for all to stop counseling and prescribing artificial contraception. Since I was still new at the clinic, it was frowned upon by some as unusual. One nurse who was a Catholic objected quite strongly to my views. But in general, the attitude of tolerance so prevalent in our society led most to accept my decision as a personal choice.

The new or old patients who came to me for advice on family planning are given information on NFP. I was surprised that many were receptive to it as many had not heard of it before, especially the non-Catholics. I also began to get referrals from patients using NFP for infertility, PMS, cervical erosions, progesterone support in pregnancy and other related conditions. It was a very gratifying experience. There is still a great deal to be learned and researched in this field. Unfortunately, very few doctors are doing it because there is not much financial support from the government let alone the pharmaceutical companies.

My experience with NFP as a family doctor was short lived. A year later, I joined the seminary with a new religious congregation, the Legionaries of Christ. Here is not the place to recount the story of my vocation. Fortunately, I managed to convince my sister who was just finishing her family practice residency program to take over my practice. She enrolled in the course to become a Natural Family Planning Medical Consultant and continued seeing and treating my patients and more referrals.

I am confident that my medical knowledge and training in NFP are not foreign to the mysterious plan of God in my life as a religious now and a priest in the future. All I can say is that I am excited to discover how this new chapter of adventure will develop itself in time.

I am a Gynecologist and she had her tubes tied

This testimony was originally written in an Italian pro-life magazine and has been translated into English. This couple is living in Ohio. They have a son and a daughter.

A few months ago, an American couple told me the story of their liberation. It was very enlightening. They had always considered themselves "normal" Catholics who attend Sunday mass plus a little bit more. He works as a gynecologist. Like almost all gynecologists, he was used to prescribing all types of contraceptives. She had been sterilized. This decision posed no grave problem; they had simply decided not to have any more children after their first and only son. "We enjoyed, and still enjoy, living well, with a certain standard" she told me frankly with a smile. Sterilization seemed to be the easiest and most definitive solution. So many couples do them.

One day, their young son came back from school. Having just learned that contraception and sterilization were wrong in his religion class, he confronted his parents — in an innocent and frank manner which he inherited from his mother. Knowing her situation, he wanted to know in all simplicity, "Why have they done it?" His parents stared at one another with embarrassment, unable to respond. That was the end of it.

At least, they had thought so. But from that moment on these two calm "good Catholics" entered into profound crisis — each one on his own without the other knowing it. "That which put me in crisis the most," he said, "is to find myself without an answer before the simple question of the kid — we did not know why we did it; we had no really good reasons nor firm beliefs. The only reason was that we did it for us!" The matter proceeded for another few long months. She was beginning to consider the possibility to have the sterilization procedure reversed. But how could she propose this to her husband? She didn't even have the courage to speak about it. Curiously, the same idea was beginning to assail his mind. But he could not imagine ever bringing this up to his wife. "And this is one of the tragedies of contraception and sterilization," she commented, "that it creates a huge wall between the spouses. Once a couple has decided not to have more children, the discussion is closed forever. Neither of them can freely speak on the subject with the other. Such an important subject for our personal lives and of the couples becomes a taboo." Thus, each of them was alone, alone in their interior crisis without the other knowing it.

One night, she was woken up from sleep by the heavy sobbing of her husband. She found him sitting on the bed bathed in tears. "Look at what we have done," he said with profound bitterness. In his hands was a copy of the short encyclical *Humanae Vitae* of Paul VI on the morality of contraception. He was given this the day before at a retreat. That night, while trying to fall asleep he began to read it out of curiosity. Instead, his sleep never came and he was awake since. Finally on that night, they were able to speak openly about the problem. They discovered with marvel that both had arrived at the same conclusion without knowing it.

So, they tried to reverse the sterilization. It worked. After a short time, they were given a beautiful and adorable daughter. He continued his work as a gynecologist, however, still giving out the contraceptives left and right. "What else could a gynecologist do?" He reasoned. Yet, after a few months, he realized that he could not do this anymore. He was aware of his moral incoherence. He decided altogether to stop giving the pill. It was a liberation — the second liberation. He knew that it would be difficult. There would not be much work for one who was not disposed to sign these prescriptions. Remember, they had wanted a good lifestyle... After many trials and journeys, he together with his wife began to dedicate themselves to letting others know the alternative to contraception that they themselves had discovered — the natural methods of fertility regulation. She commented with a smile, "It was tough, but it's worth it."

Desiring purity in our marriage

Keith has a degree in Security Administration. He is employed by a California Department of Corrections as a correctional peace officer. Christina has a degree in hotel and restaurant management. She now devotes all her time and energy to the holy apostolate of motherhood.

Keith and Christina became engaged in the spring of 1991. Admittedly, they were a contracepting couple long before the wedding day in April of the following year. Christina was wrapping up her college education in Texas. Keith had just fulfilled a military obligation in California prior to embarking on a new career in law enforcement. They were cradle Catholics and considered exceptionally "religious" by their dearest friends and family. Ironically, they are the first to confess that they were anything but the good Catholics they professed to be. Why? "Fornication," Keith answers, "also known as premarital sex, followed by the contraceptive mentality that continued to infect the first two years of our marriage."

"That tiny pill," Christina said angrily, "takes the love out of the loving. Essentially, it contradicts God's natural law by separating the procreative from the unitive. What is most tragic is that it can actually prevent a healthy fertilized egg, a conceived human being, from attaching to the uterus." "That's abortifacient," Keith said, "Like so many contracepting couples we know, we were genuinely ignorant of the dark and deadly connection between contraception and abortion." "To our knowledge," Christina continued, "the pill merely prevented fertilization. We did not understand its deadly abortifacient nature.[10] We are so thankful for God's love and mercy manifested in our lives," Christina said, "and we deeply regret that for the most self-centered reasons, such as personal autonomy and self-gratification, we consciously ignored the connection between these acts."

[10] Editor's note: Abortifacient is an agent which causes abortion. Abortion is defined as the premature expulsion from the uterus of the products of conception — of the embryo, or of a nonviable fetus. *(Dorland's Illustrated Medical Dictionary*, 27th ed.) The IUD works by creating an inflammation of the uterine wall that is not favorable for the implantation of the embryo. One of the known mechanisms of the action of the contraceptive pill is by preventing implantation through the changes of the inner lining of the uterus. (Physician's Desk Reference, 52nd Edition, 1998) Since the pill has an failure rate of 3%, it implies that ovulation can still occur in those who take the pill. The modern contraceptive pill which has a lower dose of estrogen than when it first came out, has an incidence of escape ovulation of about 25-30%. (GOLDZIEHER, JM, DE LA PENA, A, CHENAULT, CB & WONTERSZ, TB, *Comparative studies of the ethynyl estrogens used in oral contraceptives-II, Antiovulatory Potency, Am J Obstet Gynec,* 1975, 122: 619.) While there is no definitive proof that oral contraceptives cause early abortions, as pregnancy tests are not sensitive to detect pregnancy in the first week, there are many indirect proofs suggesting that they do cause an early abortion-that the lining of the endometrium is thinner, with less blood supply in women taking the pill which makes implantation difficult. (See KAHLENBORN, C., *The Oral Contraceptive Pill: Should a Christian take or dispense them?* © One More Soul, Dayton, OH, KUHAR, B, *Infant*

"It was our own sinful pride," Keith added, "that fuelled the false conviction that we knew more and knew better than two thousand years of Church teaching. It would have been much easier had we just been miraculously infused with this lifesaving knowledge before we put our fertility, the lives of our children, and our salvation at risk. It would have been good to hear about NFP in our parish."

It was not too late when they learned about the potential spiritual, emotional, physical and psychological havoc contraception can wreak on the sanctity of marriage. How did they learn? "A little soul searching," Keith explains, "and a mutual desire and willingness to live according to God's natural law. Add to that a considerable amount of prayer, a gracious supply of grace, and a good lesson in the truth which can be found in Natural Family Planning." "NFP," Christina punctuates with much conviction, "represents the truth; contraception represents the lie."

Keith describes his *conversion* as beginning with a gentle pluck on the moral strings of his heart. "I desired that my marriage to Christina be as pure and pleasing to God as humanly possible. I reflected for a long while on things that could stand some change or improvement. Contraception was at the top of the list. I shared my thoughts and convictions with Christina and asked her to prayerfully consider Natural Family Planning." Keith retrieved an NFP flyer from the file cabinet that he remembered receiving in a folder at their engagement encounter retreat. At that time, neither Keith nor Christina had the good fortune of

Homicides Through Contraceptives, Bardstown, KY, Eternal Perspective Ministries, 1997, and ALCORN, R, *Does The Birth Control Pill Cause Abortions?,* Gresham, Oregon, Eternal Perspective Ministries, 1988) What is the estimate that contraceptives act by this mechanism of preventing implantation? The standard contraceptive pill has an estimated 3% abortifacient effect. The mini-pills, which are progesterone only, have a higher probability in acting this way. The progesterone implants (Norplants) and Depo-Povera are open to a higher risk of early abortion because of a higher breakthrough ovulation rate. The "morning after pill" works primarily by affecting the uterine lining to prevent implantation. The Food and Drug Administration stated in the required text of patient information, May 10, 1977 that "IUD's seem to interfere in some manner with the implantation of the fertilized egg in the lining of the uterine cavity. The IUD does not prevent ovulation." As a further complication to the debate, there have been recent attempts to redefine conception as the moment of implantation of the embryo to the uterus. In this redefinition of conception, which has no scientific basis and is politically motivated, these powerful lobby groups try to claim that the IUD and the pill are not abortifacient. A complete treatment of this subject can be found in KISHNER CW & IRVING DN, *The Human Development Hoax: Time to tell the Truth,* American Life League, 2nd ed., 1997.

reading *Humanae Vitae* or *Evangelium Vitae*. These treasures of knowledge and faith, along with the Catholic Catechism came later as an affirmation of their decision to renounce all means of artificial birth control.

Several months passed before Keith and Christina attended an NFP introductory session. They learned a great deal in that single meeting. "For example," said Christina, "NFP couples in this modern era no longer march to the beat of the highly criticized ancient Rhythm Method." Prior to attending the introductory session, Christina told her mother of her intention to practice NFP. Christina believes it was the poor practice of the pioneer Rhythm Method that caused her mother to remark, "So, you want to get pregnant?" "The truth of the matter," Keith injected, "is that NFP is more than 99 percent accurate." Keith and Christina learned that there is no similarity between NFP and artificial birth control. "NFP facilitates an incredibly accurate awareness of *our* fertility by the presence and type of cervical mucus..." Christina continues, "with this knowledge, we can strive to achieve pregnancy or we can choose to postpone it by avoiding intercourse during that time." "It's completely natural," adds Keith, "as opposed to contraception which merely succeeds in robbing a couple of fertility along with the fruit of their fertility and any conviction of personal responsibility that accompanies each union."

Christina fondly recalls the first time that she and Keith made love with the intention of conceiving a child. "It was the afternoon on the day of our fourth wedding anniversary. We were tucked away at a romantic resort on the Big Sur Coast in northern California. Keith and I made love and were overwhelmed immediately afterward by a wonderful spell of laughter. We truly believe that it was much more than a fit of honeymoon giddiness." Keith chimes in "we believe it was the laughter of a deep interior joy predicated on our total abandonment to the will of God in our marriage. It does not get any better than that." Christina smiles, "It does not get any better than Clare, our beautiful daughter. She is God's crowning glory to our marriage... And she will have brothers and sisters!"

NFP is a precious jewel. S-P-I-C-E is a clever acronym for the Spiritual, Physical, Intellectual, Communicative and Emotional facets of NFP. This is how Keith and Christina describe how they apply SPICE in their marriage.

Spiritual — the bottom line for us is a black and white realization that we were not created to make it on our own. Our love for God, our desire to please him and our willful dependency on God is the foundation upon which all else in our marriage is built. We approach our individual and marital spirituality with a no nonsense dependency on Jesus, and on all the graces merited by his suffering and death which are so generously distributed through Mary, our holy mother. We believe that as a "Domestic church", we must remain firmly anchored through personal devotion to the Eucharist and to Mary if we stand any chance of surviving as a holy family. Christina and I attend daily mass as frequently as possible. We believe that frequent reception of the Eucharist and visits to the Blessed Sacrament for spiritual "radiation therapy" are essential. "The Eucharist", as a contemporary pope stated, "contains, in a variety of miracles, all supernatural realities". We pray the daily rosary individually and we pray the family rosary at least once a week, usually before mass. As St. Louis de Montfort wrote in *the True Devotion to Mary,* through Mary we make our total consecration to Jesus.

Physical — Keith and I are natural hand holders. That is, when we're not holding Clare or pushing her stroller. We're always holding hands whether it's a rare romantic stroll on the beach, a short walk across a big parking lot or side by side at mass. Cuddling and caressing are also expression of our love and affection. Whether we're laying one behind the other while watching a movie or falling asleep, non-genital, non-orgasmic contact is an integral physical means of expressing our love. It was not always this cut and dry. We intentionally crossed that fine line between healthy cuddling and the not so healthy, *hands-on* genital stimulation, minus the intercourse, more times than we care to admit. Simply put, we were more centered on our own gratification than we were respectful of our fertility and the purpose of marital intercourse. This challenge was particularly overwhelming and more difficult to surmount when we first began NFP.

Intellectual — the more we read about NFP, the more we learned. The more we learned, the more we understood and were able to apply the moral challenges of Christ's Church in the practice of NFP.

Communication — Open, honest communication, emotional support and creative coping are essential. Christina and I cope with the emotional ups and downs of NFP in different ways. Communicating the existence of any frustration is a good start. Leaning on the shoulders of other trusted NFP couples for emotional support is very helpful. We also try to keep each other in check by maintaining a good sense of humor. Laughing is good emotional medicine and it's a lot healthier than dragging the weight of things behind us.

Emotional — the challenges associated with NFP are frequently, at least in our experience, compounded by the normal emotional and psychological frustration experienced in the day to day practice. Variables ranging from the effects of medications, stress or breast-feeding may contribute to prolonged periods of abstinence. The good news is that the consistent practice of NFP results in the strengthening of our ability to cope with, and the subsiding of these frustrations.

"Realistically, there are moments when, depending on the regularity or irregularity of Christina's cycle, NFP can be a real cross to bear..." Keith continues, "but this cross represents the truth of God's natural law and his will as Creator and the author of all life. As Christians, we are not only obligated to carry this cross, but to promote and defend its truth by our living example. NFP is good news in the *Culture of Life*. It's the best means married couples have of countering the *Culture of Death*. That's why we persevere. How we persevere is a matter of uniting the weight of our struggles to the cross of Christ. Our Lord bears all the weight for us, except for a sliver. "It's about purity of body and soul," Christina concludes, "we do it all for the glory of God."

A difficult decision for a physician

This testimony comes from a physician who works in the Buffalo, New York area.

I began medical school in 1977 in my hometown of Syracuse, NY and did not hear much about contraception from the pulpit, whereas one learned a lot about it in medical school and during OB-GYN and Family Practice rotations. I knew that the Church had come out against contraception but had not heard much after that for a number of years. I had believed many others who told me that the teaching was "not practical" in daily life in that the use of contraceptives was lesser evil than the potential of abortion. So, with few misgivings, I followed suit and prescribed contraceptives, performed vasectomies and assisted in tubal ligations, starting in residency and continuing on thereafter. I must admit that I never liked prescribing contraceptives; it never felt like it was the right thing to do.

I always considered myself strongly pro-life and as soon as I learned about the abortion issue I was a supporter of the Pro-Life cause. I was continually annoyed to read in the magazine *ALL About Issues* (published by the American Life League headed by the wonderful Judie Brown) to hear of the abortifacient nature of the birth control pill. I wanted to think that this mechanism was not active in my patients. I even remember starting a Crisis Pregnancy Center when I was practicing in Germany with the Army. In our first meeting, one of our potential members stated that she hoped we would not address birth control in this group and I allowed that since they were separate issues that we would not address that question. I continued in this view, doing sterilizations and providing contraception without any significant twinges of conscience: save for the irritation that I continued to feel reading in successive issues of *ALL About Issues* about the abortifacient nature of the birth control pills. Judie Brown even came to Europe to assist in our training of Crisis Pregnancy counselors. I found her to be a wonderful person and I did not bring up the topic of the abortifacient nature of the contraceptive pill.

In 1987 I was transferred back to the United States to teach at a Family Practice Residency Program for the Army. While there I was put in charge of the medical student training of the residency program which included being the person to orchestrate our intern and resident selection program each year. One summer an outstanding Catholic medical student, "F.J." as he was known, came for an interview and I could tell that this was a really outstanding man. I urged him to come back and do a rotation at our hospital which he did. Many other people became impressed with him and the next year he joined our residency program as an intern. The first day that he arrived he went to the Chief of the Department and advised him that he did not and could not prescribe contraception. This came as a bit of a shock and was poorly understood by the residency director who was a very good man, but not Catholic, and unfamiliar with the teaching of the Church or the reason for it. F.J. was referred to a couple of my colleagues with whom I shared an office, both Catholics, and I chimed in with them that although I generally agreed with his philosophy that such a policy regarding birth control was not practical in modern medicine. Over the next few months I saw that he stuck to his guns and instead of having difficulties with that decision he excelled at his job and continued to provide a good witness as a Catholic physician. It was around Christmas time of that year, five months after Dr. F.J.'s arrival that the thought occurred to me as I went to confession that I had never confessed the issue of prescribing contraception. I was fortunate that my confessor was Msgr. Phil M., A very holy man who was faithful to the teachings of the Church. I walked in as a person who prescribed contraception; I walked out as a person who did not prescribe or use contraception.

The next month or two was very interesting. I read *Humanae Vitae* twice and by second time around it made a lot of sense. I related to my wife that I could no longer use condoms, having realized the sinful nature of contraception. Rather than telling me how unrealistic I was, my wonderful wife also embraced the idea, an act which I feel has strengthened our marriage tenfold. I composed a letter to send to all my patients and advised them that I would no longer be able to provide contraceptives but would help them achieve training in NFP. However, I was not allowed to send that letter and got into some hot water with my boss at work (remember, I was still in the Army). I came in contact with a wonderful woman named Mrs. Sheila S., Who was a Creighton Model NFP practitioner, in Salinas, CA. I began to learn about the Creighton Model and she began to teach NFP classes at our hospital with the sponsorship of Dr. F.J. and myself. The next year, I went to the Pope Paul VI Institute for the Study of Human Reproduction in Omaha, Nebraska, under the tutelage of Dr. Thomas Hilgers to become a NFP Medical Consultant Intern. This not only increased my knowledge of Natural Family Planning methods but also allowed me to help my patients with many of their reproductive related medical problems such as infertility, recurrent miscarriage, etc. One to two years later I left the Army and set up private practice in September of 1992 in a small town in upstate New York called Montour Falls. A woman whom I met early on agreed to go for training to Omaha and she became a NFP practitioner. She teaches NFP out of my office as well as having a private practice of her own.

I cannot tell you how much better life is since I stopped prescribing and using contraceptive. Our marriage is stronger. We have two more children: one of these was God's answer to prayers the natural way despite infertility problems, and the other was God's answer to prayer through adoption. (This provided a powerful testimony to my children of the power of prayer.) I have a wonderful practice. I am known throughout the region as the "Pro-Life Doctor" and many people drive significant distances for pregnancy and delivery or just to see a doctor who is Pro-Life. NFP information is provided to all of these patients, some of whom accept it and learn NFP. It makes for a very nice patient population, a low sexually transmitted disease rate, and a low abnormal pap smear rate, few colposcopies[11], and I have a wonderful group of patients who are like friends and family. I also will go to my grave pleased that, because of what I learned through NFP, I have been able to assist some people give life to a child when they had been troubled by recurrent miscarriage. I believe I have saved a few children through the use of hormonal methods learned in Omaha that otherwise would have died through miscarriage.

I think it is important to note that although my life changed through one act of confession and what followed from that. The seeds were planted over the years — Judie Brown and her articles documenting the abortifacient nature of the pill; my volunteer dietitian and her husband in Germany who gave my wife and me *The Art of Natural Family Planning;* the outstanding example of Dr. F. J. And of course, one faithful priest. Although I cannot reveal what was said in the confessional, I can guarantee you that he did not tell me to "follow my own conscience". I would be incomplete if I did not again mention the powerful impact that *Humanae Vitae* had on me and can have on anyone who reads it with an eye to learning the truth revealed by God through his Church. All can benefit by reading Pope John Paul II's subsequent

[11] Editor's note: A pap smear is recommended to all sexually active women where a sample of cells from the external os of the cervix is taken to look for cancer cells. Colposcopy is a procedure which examines the cervix and vagina by means of a colposcope. Both examinations are used to detect early stages of cancer in the cervix. There is a high correspondence of promiscuity and sexually transmitted diseases with the incidence of cervix dysplasia and cancer.

encyclicals such as *Familiaris Consortio,* publications by the Vatican offices such as *Donum Vitae* and *Directives for Health Care Workers,* and teachings by the Bishops on euthanasia and of course *Evangelium Vitae*, the Gospel of Life.[12] Many physicians have misgivings about not prescribing contraception, whether Catholic or otherwise. It is very common to think of the faulty idea of "the lesser evil", using contraception to "prevent abortion", and we all tend to look at our bottom line and think "how can I have a practice and not prescribe contraception?". My suggestion to those who feel that way is to follow your faith, leave it up to God, and he'll take care of the problems for you. He will. And you will be rewarded with a clear conscience, full communion with the Church, wonderful patients and yes, probably some suffering, but that just let you know that you are on the right track. Remember Our Lord suffered, and we are perfected through suffering when we offer it for his sake.

It is funny how as you grow up and become educated and feel sophisticated you tend to turn your back on the teachings of your youth. The last seven years of my life have been times of significant growth in faith and a rediscovery of many of those wonderful truths, prayers and devotions that I learned in my youth. All this because of that decision seven years ago. It came just in time too, as I have young children now and can attempt to pass that faith on to them.

In case of abnormal pregnancy

This story comes form a couple from Mississippi who has used NFP for twenty-one years. They were married in 1974 and have four children.

At twenty-five years of age, I had just completed my medical internship and I was moving to Chicago to begin a residency in Rehabilitation Medicine. I was not looking for a marriage partner (had

[12] Editor's note: See Appendix 3 for a more complete list of readings.

turned down two proposals for marriage during college) and certainly was not interested in having children. Having suffered from severe dysmenorrhea[13] since the age of twelve, I was angry with God for making me female and had sought to have a hysterectomy[14] in college but was refused because of my youth and lack of children.

Demetrios was born in Greece, the youngest of eight children, and orphaned at age two as the result of post-World War II political purging. As a street kid, he was brought to the USA by an uncle at age nine and promptly orphaned again when his uncle died two years later. He always had a strong sense of family and his biggest desire in life was a family of his own with lots of children.

At age thirty, Demetrios despaired of finding the kind of wife he dreamed of and engaged himself to a woman he did not really love so that he could at least have children. He thought better of this however, and broke off the engagement before the wedding. At that point, he made a desperate plea to God, "Send me a wife I can love for a lifetime and I will forgo what I want most in life — children."

Two years later our lives crossed, and although I turned down Demetrios' first proposal to marry and moved to Chicago as I had planned, he was persistent. Demetrios assured me that even if I were not in love with him, he would love me forever and that God had chosen me to be his wife. Six months later we were married.

We discussed children and he talked me into agreeing to have at least two, if not a half-dozen children. Since we were twenty-five and thirty-two years of age, we decided not to postpone pregnancy and used no birth control.

After one year of trying to conceive without success, I used my medical knowledge and the Couple to Couple League's handbook *The Art of Natural Family Planning* — it was introduced to me by one of my sixteen siblings — to begin charting my cycles in the hopes of achieving a pregnancy.

[13] Editor's note: Dysmenorrhea means painful menstrual cycles.
[14] Editor's note: Hysterectomy — the surgical removal of the womb.

The charting revealed that everything was perfect, 28-day cycles, five days of good quality mucus, nice temperature shifts and cervical changes. Demetrios' semen analysis was also normal. After a second year, I underwent a laparoscopy and hysterosalpingography[15] which revealed bilateral clubbed tubes: not a drop of dye would go through.

I was not too unhappy about it but Demetrios sure was. We gave up trying for pregnancy, having intercourse about two times a week without regard for my charts. Over the next four years Demetrios would sometimes express to family and friends his disappointment in not having children.

One evening, six years into our marriage, Demetrios shared with me a conversation he had with an acquaintance who suggested that he divorce me and marry someone who could give him children. He also shared with me for the first time his promise to forgo children if God would send him a good wife. "You know," he said, "I never thought that I would have to keep that promise as we both come from large fertile families. God kept his part of the bargain and gave you to me, and I plan to keep you, so I guess I'll have to accept my part and be reconciled to a childless marriage."

I was touched by this and asked for forgiveness from God and my husband for desiring barrenness. We prayed together and that month I became pregnant. On November 1980, Thanksgiving week, our son was born and we named him John, after the apostle that Jesus loved, and after John the Baptist, whose conception was a miracle.

John was nursed on demand and my cycles resumed at twelve months post-delivery. Because of our prior infertility, we choose not to try to postpone any future pregnancy God might grant. Elizabeth was born Christmas week in 1982. Again, we experienced one year of nursing amenorrhea[16], followed by three years of regular cycles with infertility.

[15] Editor's note: Laparoscopy is the surgical procedure where a fiber-optic telescope is inserted to view the internal organs of reproduction and perform microsurgery where feasible. Hysterosalpingography is a procedure where, during the laparoscopy, a colored dye is injected through the vagina to check for the anatomy of the womb and fallopian tubes. If there is no blockage, the dye should be observed leaving the fallopian tubes.

[16] Editor's note: Amenorrhea means "without menstrual flow." In her case, it is due to breast-feeding the child after birth.

By this time children had worked a conversion in me. I desired more of them. In my practice, I had stopped making referrals for abortion, putting in IUD's, and even prescribing birth control pills. The latter brought a lot of flak from both patients and my hospital employer. I was told to leave my morality out of the office, so I went back into private practice where I could be the boss. Now I was teaching NFP at the office and promoting it in the local Catholic parishes.

Demetrios at this time felt that God was calling him to keep another promise he had made while an orphan in Greece. He had promised to God that if God would look after his survival then, he would adopt a Greek orphan when he was stable, married, and financially able to handle the responsibility.

He was then forty-three and working as an attorney, married with two children. We owned our home and offices, and Demetrios felt the time had come. We figured God was calling him to his promise since our infertility was back. We underwent some studies and red tape necessary for adopting and bringing a child into the country. Our four-year-old and six-year-old were excited about the prospect of a new sibling. We had in mind a girl from two to ten years of age since infants and males would be harder to come by. We traveled to every orphanage in Greece. There were dozens of little girls, but we always encountered obstacles to our adoption. Finally I said to Demetrios, "We could adopt a disabled child, they're always available," but he would not consider it. "I would never be able to love such a child properly," he said, "I would always feel sorry for it."

We returned home empty-handed and were promptly blest with a third child, a disabled child! He was born six weeks premature with Down Syndrome. It had been a difficult pregnancy. I had gestational diabetes, chronic sinus infection and an abnormal alpha fetal protein[17].

Demetrios was devastated. He would not look at or touch the baby. He would not talk to me for two weeks except to say, "You're a doctor, you

[17] Editor's note: Alpha Fetal Protein is a blood test done to women usually over forty years of age. Its abnormality indicates the possibility of a genetic defect or abnormal child.

knew the pregnancy was not normal, you could have done something." Demetrios would not even tell me the name that he had chosen for this child so I named him Anthony, knowing that he would need a powerful intercessor in heaven.

St. Anthony came through for his little namesake and Tony gradually stole his daddy's heart. They became inseparable buddies because unlike normal children, who can be reticent, Tony loved spontaneously and unconditionally. Now, I could speak against abortion and give personal testimony to the value of the disabled.

Tony nursed for nine months during which time I was again amenorrheic. The Lord knew we needed extra time with Tony because of his medical problems and daily therapy sessions so he gave us an additional two years of unsought infertility before really putting us to a test.

When the nine months of nursing infertility ended after Tony's birth and I started cycling again, we did not avoid intercourse during the fertile time. By this time we had learned to trust that God knew what he was doing; that he would not give us more than we could handle. We had also learned to value children as the only thing of lasting worth in this life, the only thing you can take with you to heaven. In light of our past history of infertility we were not too optimistic about getting pregnant, knowing that fertility naturally declines with age.

So we were pleasantly surprised when at age forty-one I became pregnant for the fourth time. The prenatal testing indicated another Down syndrome child. I dreaded breaking the news to Demetrios but Tony had worked a spiritual conversion in his dad. Demetrios took my hand and said, "Whatever is wrong, with God's help, we can handle it."

The disapproval from society, however, was strong: "A fourth child", "at your age", "You already have a retarded child", "You can terminate the pregnancy you know". We prayed and continued to witness to the value of unborn life, however compromised. Our fourth child was born on her due date, perfectly healthy, in mind and body. She was named Mary, another precious miracle from God.

Mary weaned herself at one year of age and my monthly cycles returned at that time. It has been eight years since Mary's birth. As usual, we have left our fertility entirely in the Lord's hands since he knows better than we do what we can handle and when.

At age forty-nine, I can see by my scanty menstrual flow, shortened cycles and diminished mucus patches that I am peri-menopausal and have not the hormones to sustain a pregnancy. But then anything is possible with God if you allow him space in your life to work.

I think one of the major obstacles for couples is that they come to marriage, as I did, looking at children as a burden to be avoided instead of a gift to be welcomed. We are products of an anti-child culture. Once our hearts were converted to see children as a gift instead of a burden, pregnancy, even an abnormal pregnancy, ceased to be a problem.

Our relationship was strained while on the pill

Married for twenty-one years and using NFP for nineteen years, this couple from Ohio has four children.

We were newly married in 1976. I, Martha, am Catholic but believed that the Church had changed its teaching and allowed married couples the use of contraceptives. Ken was Presbyterian and realized that the Church still opposed their use, but as a Protestant he was willing to make full use of his wife's invincible ignorance.

After a few cycles on the pill, however, I became tired of being continuously nauseated and stopped taking the pill. We used barrier methods, but our sexual intimacy was already suffering. Then I, who was still in college, had a longer cycle than usual and became concerned that I was pregnant. I looked up "Pregnancy Centers" in the phone book to find a pregnancy test. When I called Planned Parenthood's number, I inadvertently (providentially) dialed the number on the line below, which was the Couple to Couple League's number.

Instead of receiving a pregnancy test, I talked at length with a volunteer counselor, who explained the basics of Natural Family Planning.

I became interested in using the method and talked it over with Ken. The counselor had also introduced me to *Humanae Vitae* and I realized that in conscience I could not use unnatural methods.

Ken's decision to cooperate with me was not based on religious motives. He was alarmed at the effect contraception was having on our relationship. It seemed as though contraception was a cruel taskmaster. The stress of Ken's job had reduced his sexual drive. We were living apart while I was finishing my schooling. When I returned on the weekends, it was expected that we would make love. Since I was artificially made to be infertile, there was no good excuse to abstain, even though at times Ken would just as soon not have had to "prove" his love by performing sexually. He began to sympathize with women who are forced to make love, the difference being that a man cannot fake an erection. In order to perform, he had begun using pornography.

He knew what Jesus had said about lust in the heart and realized he was in trouble. When I proposed NFP, it seemed to answer his own prayers. He had never been interested in what the pope had to say about anything, but out of curiosity he began reading *Humanae Vitae* and found that Pope Paul VI defended the Church's position on contraception brilliantly. But, beyond that, the pope's statements on the nature and meaning of marriage were beautiful truths that he had never heard before. He became more enthusiastic about NFP than me.

We became volunteer NFP teachers in 1979 and have taught continuously ever since. In our case, NFP has been 100% effective. We have never experienced a "surprise" pregnancy. After a few years of use, when Ken finally got a job with a living wage, we saw we had no sufficient reason to postpone having children. We put the method into reverse and conceived our first child. I then spaced three more pregnancies with ecological breast-feeding. The children were each between two and a half and three years apart, and each was intentionally conceived within a few cycles of the return of my fertility, which was usually about thirteen months postpartum.

Only once were we ever distressed by abstinence. My third cycle using the method was seventy-six days long. I was under a great deal of work-related stress and had a bad influenza. This postponed ovulation for two months. My mother, a registered nurse, began asking me when I would like to schedule the baby shower. No one believed that we could know with certainty that I was not pregnant. Proving to them that we were not stupid became part of our motivation to keep abstaining and not risk pregnancy with the less effective barrier methods. But we had also begun to realize the healing of our sexual relationship that comes from following God's law.

Ken was studying Catholicism by this time and had become interested in the moral theology of virtues. He began to understand that God was using this time of abstinence to teach him temperance, self-control, and that charity involves acts of sacrifice, not just emotional affection. He could see from my cycle that I was under great stress and he realized that it was his duty to console me and help me through these difficulties. In other words, the chart spoke to him and told him more about his wife than he understood from her words. We survived that difficult cycle, which both of us remember as the turning point in our relationship. Abstinence does make the heart grow fonder. We were sacrificing something important for each other, and we each knew it.

Young couples often worry that the abstinence of NFP will be a constant unpleasantness in their marriages. This is like the similar worry that renouncing contraceptives will mean having a dozen babies before they know what hit them. Neither fear is realistic. But few newlyweds have the experiences or understanding of NFP to see that they can confidently plan their family size and that there might be years of their marriage when abstinence is not needed. They seldom appreciate that their own hopes and feelings may change.

As Kierkegaard said, we are condemned to live life forwards and understand it backwards. When we began our marriage, Ken would not have welcomed the idea of having four children. Neither would he ever have dreamed that at forty-five, he would deeply regret not having started our family sooner so that we could have had six or seven children. Only through God's grace are the wishes of our youth restrained from tormenting our old age.

That elusive little pamphlet — *Humanae vitae*

This testimony comes from a couple who lives in Illinois

My story begins when my husband and I were engaged. Through my mother, I was made aware of the fact that the Catholic Church did not approve of the use of birth control. Although I was raised Catholic, I stopped attending Catholic schools in high school. I did attend CCD classes, but nothing of substance was ever discussed there. Like most twenty-two year olds, I was naturally suspicious of anything my mother told me. So we went to visit with the priest who was to marry us to find out the true teaching of the Church. Much to our relief, the priest told us that the Pope was not "talking to people like us" when he made his pronouncement on birth control. He told us that we should use our own consciences when deciding if birth control should be used in our marriage. Sadly, that was all we needed to hear. Since his position on it was much easier for us to live with, we decided to look no further.

Thank God for my mother, because she never gave up on the issue. She kept feeding me little news articles and pamphlets until I agreed to read *Humanae Vitae*. I was determined to get to the bottom of the issue even though I expected that the encyclical would be a huge volume that would take months to wade though. My mother did not have a copy of *Humanae Vitae* so I went to my local parish and asked the pastor if I could borrow a copy. Despite the fact that they had an extensive library, they did not have a copy of the teaching document. So I looked no further.

It was when a friend mentioned that she was taking Natural Family Planning classes at a local hospital that the issue finally opened up for us. Out of curiosity my husband and I went to the class. Lo and behold, there we found a copy of the elusive *Humanae Vitae*. I was shocked at its size. Instead of a massive ponderous text, it was a small pamphlet. I was even more surprised when I read it and found that it made sense.

Still not entirely understanding the Catholic Church's teaching, we finished the series of classes and began using NFP in our marriage.

God's grace continued to lead us toward greater understanding of marital sexuality. I read every book I could find on the topic, and when I was finished with that I began to wonder what other jewels of wisdom the Catholic Church contained. I began educating myself in the ways of my church. My husband followed. Our journey, which began with Natural Family Planning, left us with a sincere love and respect for our faith. My husband and I became NFP teachers five years ago. We are deeply committed to this apostolate.

As a slight aside, after accepting the Church's teaching, I went to confession and confessed the sin of contraception. In the confessional, I was told that using contraceptives was not a sin. Exasperated, I asked the priest to give me absolution just in case.

It is my conviction that discussion of the morality of contraception must center on the natural law. Today's Catholics are not impressed by something the Pope or the Magisterium says, because they have no understanding of their Church. Natural law approaches the issue from the perspective of respecting our human nature. Natural law applies to all people and not just Catholics. It outlines behaviors that are in our best interest as human beings and as a society. When natural law is viewed in conjunction with historical data from the past thirty years, it is obvious that this lack of respect for the nature of our sexuality through contraceptive use has resulted in a breakdown in the institution of marriage and families.

Our sexuality has a certain nature, and if we do not live in accord with that nature, problems will result. To determine the nature of sexual intercourse, we have to find its purpose and meaning in nature. It is obvious that the purpose and meaning in nature of sexual intercourse are babies and bonding. Babies insure the continuation of the human family and bonding creates a family structure for the raising of children. Contraception violates the natural law in that it removes the procreative aspect of sexual intercourse. We are treating the natural gift of fertility as a burden. With contraceptive use, intercourse loses its procreative meaning. The bonding aspect of sexual intercourse is also violated with contraceptive use. The marriage covenant pledges total unconditional love — unlimited commitment. With contraceptive use there is a part of our bodies that we are not sharing. There is a part of our spouse's body we are not accepting.

Similar to seeking the unitive aspect of sex without the procreative aspect in contraception, in *vitro* fertilizations seeks the procreative aspect of sex without the unitive. In both cases, natural law has been denied. With contraception, man makes himself the arbiter of when life should begin. By the same reasoning, man becomes the arbiter when life should end in euthanasia. Who would not agree that our lack of respect for the nature of human sexuality in the past thirty years has caused physical and emotional damage to our culture?

Our planning didn't work

This couple from Virginia has been married for eight years. The husband is a computer project manager while the wife is a home school mother and edits a pro-life newsletter. This testimony is adapted from an article they wrote a few years back.

Like most engaged couples, we set goals for our life together. As we progressed toward our wedding date, we constructed an ideal of what our life would be in "Our Five-year Plan." We wanted as large a family as we could afford. We anticipated three or four children, but hoped for five or six. Before having those children, we had some goals to achieve if we wanted Suzanne to stay home to raise the children. Jamie would have to establish himself in his career. Suzanne would have to finish college and establish herself in her career — just in case she ever needed it. We both wanted material "stability": money in the bank, a furnished home, and two cars. Also, we wanted to experience the pleasures of life — travel, evenings out, free living without the burden of children — just for a while. We were young, Jamie was twenty-five and Suzanne was twenty, so we had plenty of time to achieve these goals.

Our "Plan" was formed by values created by society: self-fulfillment and material comfort. The life we hoped to live was one that appeared to be easy for us and would have impressed our family, friends, and neighbors. The thought of pleasing God — by exercising stewardship over our material gains, no matter how few or many, by living a life of sacrifice, and by building a relationship with Him — as a means of fulfillment had not occurred to us. The question of when we should have children and how many we should have, was adapted to our wills in consideration of our comfort. Often, our family and friends encouraged us to postpone having children because of our young age so we could achieve worldly goals first.

After Suzanne announced our engagement to her doctor, the doctor suggested she take the pill for birth control. The doctor assumed we wanted to postpone a pregnancy for a long time; she was correct. Suzanne went on the pill. We knew that the Catholic Church prohibits the use of artificial birth control; however, we thought that meant not avoiding pregnancy at any time for any reason by any means. Our perception of living the teaching led us to envision an endless stream of children spaced nine months apart. It never occurred to us that there was a licit, effective method to avoid pregnancy, one based on God's design of the female body.

By the time we made an *Engaged Encounter,* Suzanne was experiencing some of the side effects associated with the birth-control pill. Jamie did not like seeing her suffer for the sake of "worry-free," "whenever you want it" sex.

The *Engaged Encounter* included a talk on Natural Family Planning. What impressed us about NFP was that it is an effective method of birth regulation without any side effects. We were also pleased to know it is inexpensive to use! The shared responsibility was an enticing aspect. Most of all, it was a relief to hear the Catholic Church approved of a sound method of spacing children.

The following week, we enrolled in a course taught by the Couple to Couple League (CCL) of Cincinnati. Suzanne threw away the pill, and began to feel better quickly. The first class provided us with a clear and correct understanding of the Church's teaching on sexuality and the use of contraception. We learned the beauty of sexuality when placed in the proper context. Further, we learned that birth control and sex outside of marriage can harm or destroy a marriage. We began to pray for strength in our upcoming marriage. By the second class, we had learned much about the Sympto-thermal Method. We could see that NFP is a scientific method that would work well, if we followed the method properly. By the third class, we had begun to detect the pattern of Suzanne's fertility. We planned to take the fourth class separately from the series of classes we were attending because it would be held the day after our wedding.

In looking at calendar dates and charted patterns, something occurred to Suzanne. It appeared that her next fertile time would be around the same time as class four. Meanwhile Jamie had been wondering, "What if Suzanne is fertile during our honeymoon?" He did not think it was probable. Suzanne called the wife of our teaching couple to ask, barring any physical or mental stresses, would Suzanne be fertile at about the same time in her next cycle? The answer was "probably."

We had made the decision to use Natural Family Planning by logic; however, our moral and religious convictions had grown strong. We began to realize that following God's plan for marriage means more than not sinning to avoid pregnancy, it means being generous. In order to use NFP in the proper moral context, God needed to be part of "Our Plan." We thought he was coming into the arrangement as a silent partner. We had to recognize that part of letting God into our marriage meant having him be a vocal, active partner.

We had committed ourselves, in word, to making God a part of our marriage. We would be married in the Church making our union a Sacrament and a covenant between God and ourselves. Next, we had to commit ourselves, by our actions, to the covenant among the three of us. We had to make a decision which would uphold the values which we had decided would guide our marriage. We had three choices: use contraception on our honeymoon, abstain on our honeymoon, or leave it in the Lord's hands.

We had firmly decided that contraception would have no place in our marriage. We did not want to separate the unitive and procreative aspects of the sexual act; we wanted our marital relations to be as God had intended them to be. Therefore, artificial contraception would have negated any presence of the Lord in our marriage and, thus, would have denied the values we had wanted to guide our marriage. Furthermore, pregnancy would still be possible if the birth control failed.

Abstaining on the honeymoon would have adhered to our moral convictions. Also, it would have given us complete assurance that conception would not occur. But conscious abstinence during the fertile time, without "grave motives" (*Humanae Vitae* 10), would mean refusing the Lord's offer of a child. In this sense, it would be no different from contraception. In the wedding ceremony we would be asked if we would accept children willingly and lovingly. "When we want to" was not an acceptable answer.

Thus, we had to rethink our circumstances using Christian prudence and generosity. We had already decided that we wanted our marriage to be founded on God's Plan, not ours. As the Gospel reading at our wedding would reflect, we wanted our marriage to be like the "house built on a rock." In regard to the biological laws governing fertility, we had decided that we would respect them by using NFP. Next we had to approach how we would use NFP.

Was it completely necessary to prevent a pregnancy? Were there valid reasons for avoiding pregnancy? In *Humanae Vitae*, Pope Paul VI outlined the criteria for "grave motives" to avoid a pregnancy. The couple must be limited by financial, psychological, physical, or social factors. At the same time, the couple must "conform their activity to the creative intentions of God."

We began to see the criteria by which we judged our readiness to start a family were selfish and that choosing a morally licit method of avoiding pregnancy was not enough for us to follow Christ. We could see that we were being called to abide by what was clearly God's will-for us to trust him to decide whether we had a child.

Thus, after much prayer and discussion, we chose to consummate our marriage covenant, without desecrating the meaning of the marital act, and to allow God to exercise His Will as he saw fit. Ironically, we found ourselves worried that we would not conceive. By letting the Lord have dominion over our family, we were letting him decide. We also realized he could say "no."

Although we knew that if Suzanne's temperature had risen and stayed elevated for twenty-one days and the probability that she was pregnant was 99%, Suzanne decided to have a pregnancy test as soon as possible. It was the first day of the spring semester of school, so Suzanne planned to go to the University Health Services for the test.

We agreed that we would not discuss the results over the phone; Jamie had to wait until that evening when Suzanne would pick him up at the subway station. As Jamie rode the Metro (the Washington, DC subway system), he looked around in amazement at the families that crowded the train; the train at that time of day was usually full of business people. Many of the families carried signs that read "Choose Life" and other pro-life slogans as they returned home from the March for Life. Suzanne did not need to tell him what the results were. Joshua was born about nine months later.

We had intended to space our children about two years apart. We planned to space our next pregnancy first with breast-feeding and then with NFP when Suzanne's fertility returned. When Joshua was fifteen months old, we began to take chances. We threw away the charts and decided to be open to intercourse on the outskirts of the fertile time. After a few months of not conceiving, we began to use the mucus only method to pinpoint Suzanne's fertile time without success. After six months, Suzanne went to the doctor's to find out the causes of her infertility. Ironically, the first question they asked was, "Do you have any temperature charts?"! Our knowledge of Natural Family Planning was a blessing in trying to find a reason for our infertility. Some problems were easily recognized on Suzanne's charts. She addressed these problems by nutritional changes and vitamin supplements. Also, the charts gave enough information to indicate that some tests were unnecessary.

Our understanding of *Humanae Vitae* helped us to recognize that whatever tests we pursued, they must not separate the love and life aspects of conception. Our desire for another child was balanced with our respect for the natural order, as our desire to space a birth had been. Without respect for the natural order to balance our desire, we might have resorted to immoral acts to determine the problem or to achieve pregnancy. The desire for another child had become great. Last, but not least, we are blessed to have an OB-GYN who not only understands fertility, but embraces the truth of *Humanae Vitae* and the many teachings of Pope John Paul II.

At the writing of this essay, it has been six years since we began to ask God for another child. It has been a lesson in patience that we are still learning. The few, small problems we found that could have been contributing to our infertility have been corrected for some time. Only God knows why we have not conceived.

Some time ago, a mother of seven boys gave Suzanne an insight to God's ways. The mother had said that the challenges of raising a large family had been the source of so many graces for her and her husband. Suzanne quipped that we have a long way to go because we do not have enough children. "That's not true!" Replied the mother. "God has given you *the* family that will bring you closer to him."

When we look back on our honeymoon, it is always with a sense of relief and with tremendous gratitude for the grace to be open to God's will. At the beginning of our marriage, we sacrificed material and worldly gains for the child we received. Now, we have material comfort, but we do not hold it in the same regard as we did when we were engaged. Our personal fulfillment is rooted in our humble attempt to fulfill God's will for us.

How we dealt with unexpected pregnancies

This rather long testimony comes from Missouri of a couple who has been married for 14 years. They have four children, not including the one miscarriage.

> "Do not store up riches for yourselves on earth, where moths and woodworms destroy and thieves can break in and steal. But store up riches for yourselves in heaven, where neither moths nor woodworms destroy them and thieves cannot break in and steal. For where your treasure is, there will your heart be also." (*Matthew* 6:19-21)

I was pregnant before marriage. Needless to say, our choices on sexual behavior could only change for the better. My childhood was shaped by a struggling Catholic marriage, society's loud screams of what they call *normal* behavior, and the influence of a very devout grandmother. My husband also came from a Catholic family with all their pluses and minuses. He was the older of six; I was the oldest of two.

Before getting married, we went through marriage preparation with the Church. In the classes we were given a handout on Natural Family Planning. We went over it and were told this was the Church's teaching. As we remember, almost fifteen years ago, this was presented as an "option." It was available, but not everyone uses this. Our lead couple did choose this form at some point in their marriage. We were never given a name of a teacher for any follow-up if we were interested in it.

Soon, our first little girl arrived and we were delighted with her. Hoping that we would have more children, we did not worry about the planning of another child. Just fourteen short months later, we received our son. At this time, becoming pregnant again seemed inevitable, as we were both twenty-years-old. We opted to use condoms. Albert was finishing college and working a full-time job in the produce department at a grocery store while I was a checkout clerk at another. After the first baby was born, I quit work and stayed home with the baby. We had insurance so we were able to pay our doctor bills.

At this point in our marriage we were fragile. We were very much in love but still growing up. Albert and I accepted our roles as parents well. We had tremendous support from our families. These were hard, growing times, but the Eucharist and Mass were very important and sustained us. Albert and I have always believed in the power of prayer and wanted to live as God has taught us. We were practicing Catholics on every issue except birth control.

We lived in a summer cottage that was on my parents' land. It was a wonderful home. We loved it and still have fond memories of our life together there. When our son was three months old, we outgrew our home. My parents came through with tremendous support for us for a year. They bought a home for us to rent from them. We could not pay our full rent for a year but we paid most of it and all the utilities. We felt responsible for our future and wanted not to get pregnant again. In fear we used condoms for we felt that we were doing what was socially acceptable and being responsible.

Albert went for an interview at a medical clinic for a part-time bookkeeping job. They wanted him, but he had to refuse because there were not enough hours to support our family and we needed insurance. God's saving hand interceded again. The clinic gave him everything he asked for.

One year later, my husband came home from work after running an errand to the store for milk for the babies and a few other needs. In the grocery bags were ice cream, a bottle of wine, and some other treats. I was so upset. I did not understand how he could have spent so much rationed money we did not have. I almost cried but then he sat me down and told me he was given his first real raise — a salary to support us and payments to our own home. Albert is now the vice-president of the clinic. When he started, he only worked out of a trailer. Now there are four facilities with many doctors. This is one of the many examples which shows how the Lord has loved and guided us, teaching us to trust him. Trust is a quality with which I have a hard time. Through reading the Bible, the Lord speaks to us. Many times I would come to the reading on True Riches and other readings which guided us on how to live. We would try very hard to follow them. Some lessons came easier than others did; some he is still instilling in us.

As we grew spiritually, we wanted to give back to others what God had so graciously given to us. We tried to help when needed and we became more active in our parish, community, and school. Our parish priest asked us to start a newly married couple's group. We called it *Cana Couples*. It was a group that was spiritual, educational and social. It lasted for three years. From this group we have a few couples we remain very close. We still meet and pray together, and some of us do volunteer work. Several of the couples helped us grow through their knowledge of the Catholic Church and her teachings. One of these friends was a nurse who later taught us the correct usage of NFP.

The third child was *the* child. By this I mean the child Albert and I planned. Yes, we said, with God's blessing this would be the night to make our baby. We went out to dinner, did all the romantics and planted our seed. The next month followed and we were happy to make our doctor's appointment. The doctor did an ultrasound. I was thrilled with the procedure because I could see our baby curled up in the cradle position at the bottom of the screen. Not thinking anything was wrong, the doctor said, "Ann, the picture is not right." He continued, "There is no motion on the screen from the heart, there is no heartbeat." I had a cold feeling come over me and was in shock. What did I do wrong, thinking that I am so healthy and young? He explained that this is quite common and that most women experience miscarriages. He wanted me to have a D&C (Dilatation and Curettage — the scraping of the walls of the womb) but I did not want it. He agreed to see if my baby would pass naturally and it did.

I will never forget that morning. I woke up feeling I was ready for labor but reality hit seconds later when I remembered that this baby was dead. We went to the hospital that night and the ward was very full. I even had to share my room. The doctor was as patient as he could, but said that I only had so much time to finish the delivery. He was probably stressed out for time with so many other babies arriving. The labor was just like giving birth with all the contractions. We could hear women screaming, the fetal monitor next to us in the room, and the cries of babies' first breaths. It was overwhelming and left an emptiness which we cannot describe.

This experience drove home that life is more than genetics, and we are not in control. It is God's intervention and truly a very special gift. The doctor came in at the last five minutes. We said a little prayer and my body responded. I was able to push the baby out. At that time we did not know what to do. How developed was the baby? We knew they could not tell us the sex. We would have had some type of funeral service knowing and feeling the way we do now. This event took me a few years to get over. I did not want to replace that baby with another. We had two beautiful children and were happy. In fact when looking back I think the spacing between our children and the loss of the third baby was a time for personal development.

Five years later, my two children were close to being in school full time and I was prepared to go back to school. We were not using any contraception but we followed the calendar method (Not the true NFP method we now use). So, when I became pregnant again, there was some readjusting in my thinking. Yet we were very excited to have another baby. We were more mature and less nervous about being perfect parents, knowing that we could only do our best and pray. Our prayers have always been answered for the best. We were learning the full meaning of "God's will be done" in our lives and accepting it.

After our third baby was born, we went through our first NFP classes. We thought we knew it but not well enough. Our teacher was very good. We got to know her and her husband through our *Cana Couples* group so we were a little uncomfortable to share our private life at first. Trust is a big thing for me and I will not just talk to anyone. The teacher was very professional and had her associate RN degree which assured us that she knew what she was doing. This helped us to be less embarrassed. She was extremely repetitious, which drove me nuts but which drilled into me confidence. She neither taught nor accepted anything outside the rules. She also had a very compassionate understanding of our trials with this method. This was not just a religious issue or a part time job for her.

We both learned many things from our teacher. I can now interpret the signs of my body. I learned how to chart according to my cycle and not the calendar. While I do the observations, Albert is in charge of charting. Not all couples do this but we prefer this so that we share the responsibility. There is not just one taking responsibility as in having to wear a condom or taking a pill. It's nice for my husband to see where I am in my cycle and understand how I am feeling. This method is very comfortable in that we enjoy actual contact with each other without interference of any man-made substances that take away personal bonding. This is natural and feels very right. At the time of abstinence, we court each other. In this "I want it now, when I want it" society, I'm afraid that couples are missing out on the fun of courtship within their relationship. I'm talking about time with each other — playing games, doing things you like, talking, relaxing and, most important, praying together. These are times when you see all the qualities that attract you in the other person or areas where there is room for growth together. It is good to discover them again before potential problems arise.

It is not always rosy. Albert works many hours because the clinics are open 365 days a year until eight in the evening, and the doctors have meetings after this. Late nights are common. I have to keep the household going all by myself for the most part. I try very hard to enhance the children's education at home and both have music lessons among the many other activities. Our lives are very full and when we have non-fertile times to be with each other, we are often exhausted or activities keep us apart. When I was nursing, my cycle would be irregular. Not wanting to become pregnant we would have to abstain sometimes up to six months. During days of fertility or irregular cycles, we would avoid each other by becoming busy. I would become cold and push away any affection Albert would show me. Albert would have to suppress himself for so long that he would become cold, too. It was lonely and hard for both of us. But with prayer, God helped us through these times. We thought that this was to make up for the times we did not abstain before marriage. From this we felt as if we were purifying our marriage. We also look on these times as a kind of cross to carry, but a small one to offer for all that God has done for us. Now during our non-fertile periods on special days or holy days, we sometimes offer them up as sacrifices.

Five more years later the three children were all in school full time. I wondered what I should do next. Albert and I talked it over and we decided that we'd see how the year would go with me at home. I was thinking of getting a part-time job or go back to school to study real estate or pharmacy. But at the same time, we felt a great void in the thought of not ever having a baby again in the house. We were twenty-nine years old. Some people were just getting married. We were still full of life and this seemed to be a waste of our fertility and vitality. So we waited for signs from God but did not receive any so I was ready to begin a more personal life for myself. But be it job or school, I had to be there whenever the kids were home. Family always comes first.

Well then, of course I became pregnant again. I was overconfident in our charting and my observations that it almost felt like a safe piety. Boy oh boy, was I frustrated! I started to take it out on my teacher, but looking back at everything it was so obvious it was not her fault, she told us all the rules. Then whom could I blame this? I thought, "Okay, Lord, I have been a good girl, doing what you say I should. I even lived my sex life in accordance with your teachings and we went for our further education. I gave you time to respond to my request. Now that I decided to have more freedom for myself, you give me another child. What's the pay off here?"

Reality was, I still wanted to be in control and wanted God to answer my request on my time line. Was I truly open to life? Or was I only using NFP as a moral contraception, so I could live my life with a clean conscience. I still really thought I was the one in control as long as I followed all the rules. I realized that I had not used NFP with a true openness to life. After I got through my anger and resentment stage with prayer, God helped me to heal and understand. I was able to accept the fact that NFP was a openness to life and that really we had little control. I accepted the fact that at any point while practicing NFP we could conceive again. NFP is being open to life not another form of birth control. We stopped calling non-fertile times "safe time". Those non-fertile times are still times to be open to God as well as the fertile ones. To accept children was apart of our marriage vows and commitment to each other and God. A daughter was born one day before my thirtieth birthday.

When she was a year and a half old I became pregnant again with our fifth child, our fourth daughter. We were happy at the thought of another sweet baby and I was glad they were close in age. I did not want another five year break. I had already had the children in school full time twice. To taste personal freedom twice and start all over was tough.

This time my stage of growth was to rely on God totally, and to accept yet another child. I did not feet I could go through another pregnancy and felt my body was tired enough. Yes, I knew God was present in the conception of life and this was his plan. Yes, I knew all children were blessings. Yes, God I love little babies, but five! I do not even have the energy to go through another pregnancy let alone lying on that table to deliver again. How do I deal with this? My heart responded, "Ann do you love me? Ann you do and you are obedient and loving. But you have not given me your full trust, your heart, and your full being. You must die to yourself and let me in your life. Well now it's time, Ann, to educate your soul and mind and truly accept life in your heart and not only in obedience to my will."

I went through a year and a half of wonderful healing and growing experiences. My husband and I went on *Cursillo* weekends and other retreat weekends at Conception Abbey. I held my *Cursillo* cross all during my delivery, which was a healthy natural delivery. When the nurse tried to take my cross out of my hand so that I could hold the grip delivery handles better. I fought with her to leave it alone.

Finally, I truly have acceptance in my heart and I thank God for this grace. Albert had all his worries and concerns, as a man would, to provide for us. Still he was always joyous and was full of acceptance for the children God faithfully sent us. I already was given the most important need from God. I was given a devoted, loving and prayerful husband. When worries arise I still occasionally open up to the passage on the True Riches which puts a happy smile on my face. Yes, Lord you have always provided for us. Thank You!

With each child God has taught me many things, not only with the pregnancies but also with the temperament of each child. I would go to heaven not by myself alone but through my children and husband. I'm sure we have many more trials to grow through, but this is but a small example to share with you. There were many other little lessons too numerous to share in our use of NFP.

The Good News of Natural Family Planning

From Sacramento, California, this couple has been married for four years. They have recently conceived a son. He works as an auditor and she works as a budget analyst.

We had been married for two years when we started "toying" with NFP. I heard of it from a friend and bought a book written by one of the pioneers of NFP — Dr. Billings. I was embarrassed to ask anyone how to use NFP so I wanted to learn it on my own. I read the book from front to back several times. I thoroughly looked at the instructions, made "visual" observations, charted them and used the method. We used it for three months before seeking "professional help" from the Mercy Women's Center in Sacramento, California. I had thought that NFP was a lot of work, but spending time with my instructor and learning how to use it dispelled this misconception.

The reason why we switched from the pill to NFP was because we wanted to see if it really worked. We did not have any children and thought, well, it does not work for avoiding pregnancy, we'll just have one kid and know that it does not work. Well, it works! It has been 100% effective for us — as long as we make good observations and charts and follow the rules.

We do not have any children now and now we are planning to use it to plan a family. We chose NFP because it uses no chemicals, and requires not one partner to bear the responsibility of birth control — it is a shared responsibility. This solved our problem of the pill and the vasectomy. Besides, NFP is different from contraception promoted by the Planned Parenthood in that it is natural. It is awesome to see the daily changes in the mucus of my body. NFP does not change what God has given you. God is truly the Creator of all things.

God is and should be the foundation of our marriage. We strive to serve him daily in our lives by being living witnesses for him. In addition, we serve weekly at first and second grade Sunday school and participate in a weekly Bible Study fellowship.

Periodic abstinence may seem difficult at first, but it makes sex worth waiting for! It also helps to have good communication — we discuss problems that we may be facing and are taking a class together so we bounce a lot of info off each other daily. Also, we workout together about three to four times a week inside the gym or outside jogging. What make NFP work is God and communication. Our daily dependence is on him for all our needs.

We love NFP and have told our friends. My sister is getting married and will be using it. Her future husband supports it. I always carry NFP brochures of future classes, just in case someone is interested. The way I go about praising NFP, you'd think I am on commission!

Postscript: We have successfully used NFP to start our family. In July 1998, we were blessed with a healthy baby boy. His name is "Abraham Silas" meaning "friend of God" and "faithful one." NFP not only can enable successful conception but also determine the gender. God truly is the father of lights and gifts. (*James* 1:1) My sister got married in July 1997 and has been using NFP effectively.

Chastity what? It blew our minds

The following article is a newspaper clipping from the Archdiocesan newspaper of Hartford. Here is how Archbishop Whealon introduced the article, "Recently a national Catholic weekly published a powerful letter to the editor. Using ideas and language that no priest could think of, the author described her difficult journey to chastity." Here is the letter.

Though my hands are full with three children and with work outside the home as retail clerk, I feel moved to write in defense of the sexual sensibilities of those millions of us who are not Ph.D.'s or DRE's or [Phil] Donahue dissent superstars or even wannabe's.

YES, I was alive and fertile in 1968. I was 19 and I *knew* the pill was a gift from God and *Humanae Vitae* was a real crock. The pill was going to eliminate teenage pregnancy, martial disharmony and world population problems, bring a new era, etc.

By my five-year high school reunion, those of us who had been so confident about contraception had gone from euphoria to anger. Nothing seemed to work. I'd been on the pill less than two years before I'd quit. The pill depressed us. Or scared us (especially those of us who were smokers) because of the "stroke" factor. I did not want to keep taking it year after year, or on-again off-again after I broke up with my college lover. So I decided to live a minimally healthy lifestyle and quit both smoking and oral contraceptives.

The 'safer' IUD (copper T) gave me cramps and heavy periods. I was lucky. A friend of mine got such a ghastly infection from her IUD she lost her uterus, tubes, ovaries — the works. The woman was devastated. She felt like a gutted shell. Now they have taken them all off the market.

I tried the diaphragm. Hard to keep motivated on that one... I felt wadded up with junk, inwardly disgusted. I wanted to be delectable, like a Haagen Dazs ice cream cone; instead I was a spermicidal sump...

By the 10th high school reunion, my friends were still fiddling with this method and that, they'd had abortions, and/or their marriages were falling apart. Mine almost did.

Then my husband and I settled on the condom plus periodic abstinence. But we depended on the condom in a way that made it easy to rationalize some 'fudging' on abstinence. ("I'm probably fertile, but hey, we have got the ol' rubber so what harm can it do?") You know what 'fudging' can lead to. Thank God I did not have an abortion, but I did have one heck of an untimely pregnancy.

Finally, my husband and I reached a turning point. At a very low point in our marriage, we met some great people who urged us to really give our lives to the Lord and to be chaste in our marriage.

That blew our minds. We thought it meant 'give up sex.' That's not what it means. It means respecting bodily union as a sacred act. It meant acting like a couple in love, a couple in *awe,* not a couple of cats in heat. For my husband and me, it meant Natural Family Planning with no rubber, no 'fudging.' And I will not kid you. It was a difficult discipleship.

NFP and a chaste attitude toward sex in marriage opened up a new world for us. It bonded my husband and me in a way that is so deep, so strong, that it's hard to describe. Sometimes it's difficult, but that makes us even closer. We revere each other. And when we do come together, we're like honeymooners.

Sad to say, I was past 35 when I finally realized that the Church was right after all. Not the grab your-sincerity-and-slide church of Charlie Curran, but the real Church, the Church we encountered through lay people in the Couple to Couple League, the *Catholic* Church. The Church is right about contraception (it stinks), right about marriage (it's a sacrament), right about human happiness (it flows-no, it *floods* when you embrace the will of God). It gave us depth. It opened our heart to love.

This is why Natural Family Planning should be taught in a general way in every marriage course in a Catholic high school, and in a specific way to every couple preparing for marriage.

A difficult Church teaching turns out to be a precious jewel

This couple from Texas has been married for ten years. They have four children. They have been using NFP for ten years. The husband works as an airline pilot and the wife stays at home looking after the kids.

During our engagement to be married, Jenny and I stumbled upon one of the jewels of the Catholic Church. We graciously accepted the gem, but we carried it for years without understanding it's immense value. As we carried the treasure through our new life together, we sometimes felt its weight. We thought that it became burdensome, and we began to regard it as some millstone, rather than the precious jewel that it is. Occasionally, we even set this treasure aside, considering its small weight to be too heavy to carry any further. Those times were dark, without the shining radiance of our jewel, but we were blinded to the simple truth that the darkness was caused when we shut out the light. Well, we wandered through the darkness, and by God's providence, we stumbled back upon the beautiful jewel that we had set aside. We lifted it back up, and we were amazed in two ways. In studying our jewel, we found that it had more beauty than we had ever realized. Then, as we carefully guarded the brilliant treasure, we discovered that it felt far lighter after studying its beauty. We could no longer hide our brilliant gem under a bushel basket, we felt compelled to place it on a lamp stand so that the entire household could share in the jewel's radiance.

So, just what is this valuable gem? I am sure that many have correctly concluded that I am referring to the Church's teaching on contraception. For many, this is the most difficult teaching of the Church. With just a little understanding, though, it can be seen as the shining jewel that I describe above. I intend this article to be part of our placement of that jewel on a lamp stand.

To begin, we must first know what the Church really teaches about contraception. As most of our Protestant brothers and sisters abandoned centuries of shared belief, that contraception is against God's will, Pope Paul VI was called upon to clarify the Catholic position. After much study and debate, he released the encyclical *Humanae Vitae*. There he acknowledges that sex has an important unitive value for marriage, as well as having a procreative value. He rightly teaches though, that God has combined these two aspects into the marriage act, and it is not our place to separate them. He goes on to tell us that the unitive value is important enough that it is completely acceptable for a couple to time the marital embrace so that it coincides with the naturally infertile part of the woman's cycle, if there are sufficiently serious reasons to avoid or postpone pregnancy. He goes on to challenge Christian men of science to define more clearly the natural patterns of fertility and infertility.

Today's Natural Family Planning is the result of that scientific study, and our purpose is to let all know what a wonderful enrichment NFP has been for our marriage. In real experience, we can say that NFP builds good communication and cooperation, and that these traits are essential to any good marriage. So, in developing these traits by using NFP, we actually enhance the entire relationship. Statistically, couples using NFP have less than a 6 percent divorce rate, while the US population as a whole has a rate of 50 percent. Respecting the natural combination of the unitive and the procreative aspects of sexuality seems also to follow Father Kentenich's organic philosophy of life Contraception, on the other hand, exemplifies the mechanistic separation of what truly belongs together.[18]

We knew these things even when we occasionally succumbed to the temptation to use contraception. So what is different now? I am not exactly sure, but I know that it is associated with the conception and birth of our third child. Jenny miscarried, in the month before Adeline was conceived, so perhaps we came to better understand the fragile nature of God's gift of life. Also, in knowing when ovulation occurred for those pregnancies, we felt a warm partnership with our Creator, as opposed to the cold feeling that we felt as we placed barriers between

[18] Father Joseph Kentenich (1885-1968) is the founder of the worldwide Schoenstatt apostolic movement. He studied and developed the concept of mechanistic thinking and its antithesis, organic living. This article was originally written for a local publication of the Texas province of Schoenstatt International.

ourselves and the Eternal Father. With Adeline's birth we just knew that we had to embrace NFP completely, and we knew that we should learn to teach NFP, so that we could pass this gift on to other couples.

The Couple to Couple League accepted us as a candidate teaching couple. After about a year of study, we were certified to teach NFP. Now we offer classes at our parish, and we wholeheartedly welcome all interested couples to attend. Please keep in mind that it is not only effective, but is also reversible. NFP offers a number of "low tech" helps that many couples with marginal fertility have used in achieving pregnancy.

Practicing NFP can seem very difficult in a society that revolves around sexual gratification. We can extract ourselves though, from this collective way of thinking. With NFP, we learn to respect the whole person of our spouse. Then we can know and live the words of the Lord, "My yoke is easy, and my burden light." (*Mt.* 11:30).

Unplanned Pregnacy

Married for nineteen years, this couple from Florida has been using NFP for fifteen years. They have four children aged five to fifteen. He works as a utility manager and she is a homemaker.

The wife speaks:

We have been married nineteen years. At the beginning we used the pill but it did not agree with me so we went to condoms and foams. I had a Catholic school upbringing through high school and felt guilty about the contraceptive use, but we did not know there was anything else out there. We knew that "Rhythm" did not work. My parents conceived me while they were using Rhythm. There was a wedge in between us about the whole thing. I also felt angry that a bunch of guys in skirts were dictating to me the way I should live.

We were married about two years when, while visiting a nun from our parish, we noticed a book about Natural Birth Control from an organization called The Farm. It was like the answer to a prayer. Now we were able to live within the guidelines of the Church without guilt and we felt better about it and ourselves. We started using it almost immediately. About a year later we were introduced to the Couple to Couple League by another couple in our parish and got the book and learned the method from the book. It was a much more thorough book than the first. We have been using it ever since. We have been teaching the method for 10 years.

We feel that through NFP, God still has a door that he can work through us. All our children except for one were planned. The second was a "surprise," but in reviewing our charts, we realized that her conception should not have been totally unexpected. At first I was angry because I did not think I was ready but she is a very special child, an individual not like any other person. It was a growing time. When we first married, I only wanted one child but God had other plans. I was able to open up and it prepared me for the four I now have. When people ask if I'm finished (as if it's any of their business), I say, "I don't know."

The husband speaks:

Although I was willing to go along with my wife's desire to use NFP, I was inwardly rebellious at first, and questioned whether NFP was really the right thing to do. It seemed to be causing a lot of tension in my life and in our marriage. I am glad that we continued with it though, because I eventually realized that the tension was due to the conflict between my selfish desires (regarding sexual intercourse) and the basic Christian teaching of unconditional love. It took me years to identify the extent of the conflict and overcome the doubts about the method and lifestyle. There is so little support for NFP in this country that on a daily basis, we often feel alienated from our friends, from our acquaintances, and even from our church community on this issue.

I believe any married couple with young children experiences less sexual spontaneity than was the case before children, so this is not something I can blame on NFP. Children are just so demanding on our time and energy that we do not have the inclination for as much "spontaneity" as when we were first married. I could see where this might be difficult for a newlywed couple to live with. Many couples in our culture like to establish their careers, households, lifestyles, or relationships before they have children.

Spacing children with breastfeeding

From New Jersey, this couple has been married for six years. At the time of writing this, they have three children — Kayla age four, DJ age two and Daniel seven months. He works as a general contractor and she is a registered nurse. They have used NFP for the last five years of their marriage.

We first heard of NFP during a twenty-minute brief in *Pre-Cana*. Unfortunately, it took almost one and a half years into our marriage before we realized how evil contraception was. Yes, I was on the "pill" — unknowing of the abortifacient property and devastated when I realized the truth. Praise God for my mother. She met a woman in North Carolina practicing NFP (Sympto-thermal Method). From there we have had three planned pregnancies using NFP. I have adopted the natural breast-feeding and am spacing children with this God given means. People ask, "Why so many children and so quickly? Do you want more?" The answer is *yes* to both. When you open your life to God, the love is so overflowing. Parenthood becomes a blessing and no longer a chore. Each life that God bestows us with brings forth more love and, oh, such joy. Our children are such priceless jewels-precious gifts to us. In God's time we will have more.

As far as abstinence is concerned, this is the key to our successful marriage. It is a time of loving, giving, cuddling — bringing us closer in communication and gives us time to grow closer to God — in prayer together. No longer is our relationship focused on the sexual act. We are focused on God and then each other. Also, a time of abstinence keeps the sexual act, always something to cherish and exciting. In closing, we are becoming NFP instructors. God wants us to spread the word.

NFP helped me to recognize a miscarriage

Married for twenty-two years, this couple from Los Angeles has five children aged from twenty-one to seven. They have used NFP for fif-

teen years. The father is an operation foreman, whereas the mother is a home maker and works in child care.

When I first heard about Natural Family Planning, I was scared that it would not work. In the Pre-Cana classes, nothing was really mentioned about this very important subject although I knew this is what the Church taught about planning our families. The Rhythm Method was skimmed over and not given any serious consideration as a means to live our faith out obediently. I was told that if you have intercourse without some types of protection such as a condom, or the pill or some other birth control device you would get pregnant.

We regularly went to church Sunday after Sunday. But both of us had finished our catechism in about the fourth or fifth grade. And that was the extent of our religious training. After receiving Baptism in the Spirit I began to grow spiritually.

It was not a completely holy decision to begin the practicing of NFP. A yeast infection for almost a year led me to seek another method of birth control — we were using condoms and it was so painful for me. When I read the book *The Art of Natural Family Planning,* I thought, "these people are Christians and they wrote a book about it, so it must work." The book was very easy to read and I understood almost everything.

In my heart I knew this NFP was the right thing to do. As I read the book, it completed my knowledge of chastity I had known as a young person. This was the way to remain pure in the way we treated each other and respecting our God given procreative abilities. My husband was not as convinced as I was because of the abstinence involved, although he was not totally against it.

We continued to live in our sin for a few more years using contraceptives because I had not learned how to say no while we were dating. We were both influenced by our culture at the time because it seemed that everybody was doing it.

After my husband had a seizure, we felt it was important to live in obedience to the Church's teaching. If we were to die, we wanted to be ready to meet our Maker. We had to decide if we were being open to what God wanted in our lives. If we had so much trouble with abstinence, maybe God was calling us to have another child. We did not think it was wise for us to seek a pregnancy because I had a really tough time at the birth of our fifth child and my husband was having health problems. We had a trial month after abandoning ourselves to God's will in our life. Through God's grace, we went through a period of about three years not conceiving and yet being open to new life.

Then it happened. I became pregnant. It was kind of hard for us to accept at first because we were concerned about what the future would hold concerning our health. The whole family was afraid I might die this time because I came real close to death at the birth of our fifth child. I was not concerned the way I thought I would be. I was putting everything in God's hands. This was his child and he would show us the way. It took my husband longer to accept the pregnancy. I guess it is because his body does not have the hormones that a mother has which helped me accept it more readily.

I told my husband there are two ways we could look at this. We could be sad that we did not get our way; or we could be joyful and anticipate the wonderful baby that God was giving us as a gift. Children are gifts from God and we both love children.

The doctor kept wanting to do some tests first because of my age. She told me that I had one chance in thirty of having a baby with a deformity. At my first office visit, an ultrasound was done to see the size of the baby. She scheduled another ultrasound appointment two weeks later because of my age. Then she said the baby was not growing the way it should be and so I had to come in for an ultrasound weekly. I refused to have any test other than ultrasound because I knew this was God's gift and that we were going to love this baby, even if it were deformed or had health problems. We would not abort.

With my knowledge of NFP I was aware of my body's signs and could sense that the pregnancy might not go to term. I kept having cold spells, which was an indication that I was about to have my period. I went on a healing retreat and asked for the healing of my baby and myself. On that retreat I began the process of a miscarriage. The night before I had the miscarriage, I had a dream that the baby was a boy. I was able to see him. We named him Matthew which means gift of God.

I am thankful because I knew I could have conceived about three years prior to this pregnancy and that I had not because of NFP. So I feel sure that this is a child God wanted us to have but also that he wanted to take him home with him. Although this was an unplanned pregnancy, it was no surprise. We had about two other unplanned pregnancies while on contraceptives but they, too, were no surprise. These were our yes to God and acts of obedience.

My husband and I believe we are called to continue practicing Natural Family Planning more conscientiously and that we must follow the rules if we expect it to work. We also feel pretty sure now that God wanted our yes to his will in our lives.

The periodic abstinence has affected our life for the best. We are kinder and sweeter to each other while we are in the waiting period. Please pray for us that we may continually be open to God's holy will in our lives.

Irregular cycles and fears of pregnacy

Married for twenty-nine years, this couple has used NFP for twenty-four years. They have four children. Living in Tennessee, the father works in construction, whereas the mom is a social worker.

We learned about NFP in September 1975 when a visiting priest, who later became the Family Life Director of Owensboro, Kentucky, visited our parish to tell the congregation of the upcoming series to be taught. The class began in February 1976. Sherry had been taking the birth control pill for four years and decided to stop taking it. We were concerned about whether NFP could be used with her very irregular cycles. Variation in cycle lengths had been twenty-six to eighty days in the three years previous to the starting the pill. We decided to start NFP out of sheer desperation to learn more about natural methods of family planning, because our doctor could not seem to help us with further information.

The cycle irregularity did not change when Sherry stopped the pill, but with NFP we learned how to use the irregularity to our advantage to have more free periods of intercourse without the "fear" of pregnancy. We are very straightforward that if anyone claims that they cannot use NFP because of irregular cycles. We have a great testimony for that!

We began the practice of NFP with a contraception mentality. We wanted no more children. Years later we had two births spread eight years apart. The second pregnancy was a "Day 6" dry-day pregnancy. We did not plan it, but God had better ideas for us than we could ever have imagined when he gave us this beautiful child.

Periodic abstinence has been a benefit to our lives. Otherwise we could (and maybe would) have saturated our lives with only physical interests in each other. The time that we are apart physically has been an opportunity to grow together emotionally

We began to teach NFP after the first year of practicing it. Our twenty years of teaching through the Couple to Couple League have brought us immense growth and spiritual development. Seeing other couples grow after they learn NFP has strengthened our own marriage.

Natural and greater peace of mind

He is a manager and she works as a library director; this couple from Wisconsin has used NFP for sixteen years of their twenty-three years of marriage. They have three children aged fifteen, ten and six.

I learned about Natural Family Planning from my older sister six years into our marriage. For one month, we took a class in a neighboring town (this is very rural country) but "failed" the class because I became pregnant after the third month going off the pill.

Still, I decided to continue using NFP because it is a method which keeps in practice with my faith. I attribute this decision mostly to the prompting of the Holy Spirit.

NFP is a partner in nature. It allows us to know the timing of conception and it reveals the wisdom of the workings of our reproductive system. It provides the way for parenting that God wants us to be.

Despite this first pregnancy after going off the pill, NFP has been very effective for us. My cycles are consistently twenty-five days, with very evident mucus patterns that we do not need to take temperatures. We broke too many thermometers in the beginning anyway. Natural mothering — family bed, breast-feeding until the ages of three or four — spaced my cycles so I could not get pregnant for the two to three and a half years after birth of a child.

The periodic abstinence is getting more difficult in middle age than it was when we were younger. At that time we were so very busy with care of the children and amenorrhea for extending periods while breast-feeding made it simpler. Now with more time on our hands and decreasing hormones it is almost nature's call to push to reproduce. My husband has a much more difficult time, so we caress a lot since we avoid any coitus in Phase I also. Keeping busy and Christ-centeredness diminish impulsive sexual behaviors as we become in more control.

NFP is a blessing to our marriage as it gives a definite direction in all aspects of our functions as parents or parents-to-be. Responsible, accountable, people-directed rather then self-directed, it emphasizes the cooperative nature between a couple. My husband always knows what day it is of my cycle. But even if he knows that timing is all-important, the woman still has the main responsibility. He also understands that if I have a PMS episode, my hormones are to blame rather than me. My husband has given a witness at a premarital conference about how NFP has worked for us.

After being on the pill for more than six years, I find that NFP has brought me more peace of mind. We can live without the emotional, spiritual and physical problems of determining the number of children we will have according to our own wishes rather than the Lord's. In this world, it is easy to put yourself first rather than love. NFP makes an enlightened choice for our destiny as parents. Children have more advantages in this decision from the beginning as they are created in God's will and their whole constitution is geared toward that love source. Without having to stress loving and sharing with my children, I have noticed these characteristics in their personalities. (No, they are not *perfect* children.)

Messing with the regulators of reproduction will have its repercussions. Nature usually cannot be cheated without its effects being felt in this generation as well as future ones. And I have no problems talking abstinence with my teenage children because it is a regular part of my life as well as their dad's.

Healthy, effective and it saved her life

Married for sixteen years, they have use NFP for 13 years and are blessed with four children. They live in Ohio and the father works as a research scientist while the mother stays at home as a homemaker.

Even though Carmen had sixteen years of Catholic education, when she was to be married she did not have an accurate understanding of the Church's teaching on contraception. Phil was not Catholic at the time. We knew there were some significant health risks associated with "the pill" and the intra-uterine device (IUD) so we chose to use barrier methods in the beginning of our marriage. These, however, caused Carmen to experience chronic urinary tract infections. We soon felt that God was leading us to begin our family. After the birth of Christopher, Phil entered the Rites of Christian Initiation of Adults (RCIA) program. It was during that time that a young priest at our parish began talking to us about Natural Family Planning. We were both very skeptical initially and were convinced that it did not work (we were thinking rhythm). He suggested that we read *Humanae Vitae*. That was a turning point, especially for Phil.

We were definitely looking for something that would suit us especially in terms of health. We took a class on NFP and were quite amazed at how simple and effective it was. During the course of that first series we became pregnant (planned) and we decided to become a teaching couple. It was a dead heat between Beth's birth and receiving our certification.

Even though we were originally "sold" on the health aspects of NFP, through the years we have come to an even greater appreciation of its other benefits that God in his infinite wisdom has built into the fertility system.

One aspect of NFP that has been a great help during our marriage is that of abstinence. Learning how to cope with abstinence in small amounts when using NFP makes it much easier when longer times are necessary. These extended periods are common for most couples around the time of a new birth. We have also experienced long periods of abstinence due to Carmen's surgeries and Phil's transfer overseas.

As a research scientist, Phil had to relocate in late June one year. At this time Carmen was pregnant. The three kids and he had to stay in the States, awaiting the birth of number four. In mid-August, Stephanie was born. Phil made it home for her birth but had to return soon after. The rest of the family followed at the end of September. During this assignment, Carmen and Phil were separated for eight weeks. These were trying times but because abstinence was already part of our lives, these long stretches did not add significant stress.

We tell couples that NFP is not only healthy to use but that in our case it probably saved Carmen's life. Fourteen months after the birth of our third child and breast-feeding, Carmen's fertility appeared to be returning. Around this time, we took a bit of a risk one cycle. Since Carmen experienced a period a few weeks later, we did not think she was pregnant. However, over the next seven weeks very strange signs were observed, signs of being both fertile and infertile at the same time. Carmen's physician thought that she had a luteal cyst which would eventually rupture and things would return to normal. He even suggested that she went on the pill to see if things would get back to normal quicker. Carmen could not handle the thought of being on the pill, even for therapeutic reasons. So we waited.

Two days before Christmas, Carmen's abdominal pain became very intense. Because of our practice of NFP and having a very good handle on what is normal, we were much more insistent to the doctor that there was something terribly wrong. So, her doctor suggested a pregnancy test just to be sure. The test was positive. She was admitted immediately to the hospital and her tubal pregnancy burst through the fallopian tube on the operating table. We truly feel that had we not been using NFP, Carmen very well might have died because this all happened on a big holiday weekend and death is not uncommon for tubal pregnancies.

As we are getting older and in the early stages of pre-menopause, we are better able to understand the physical changes that are taking place as well as some of the accompanying emotional changes. As the hormones begin to decline, so does some of the interest in sexual intercourse. It is easier to see why so many couples do not make it through the "mid-life crisis." As an NFP couple we have had many years of practicing to say, "I love you" in non-sexual ways. Hence, both of us understand this as a prelude to another chapter in our lives and not a loss of interest in each other.

Not always so easy — my husband had a vasectomy

I am a Registered Nurse who works part time in an Intensive Care Unit. I am attracted to the maternal-child area of nursing and will consider graduate education at some time. I am discouraged to know that a Catholic education and practice maybe far out of reach. There are probably less than a hundred doctors involved in Natural Family Planning who give primary care to women of childbearing age.

I learned about NFP first from an article in the Sunday newspaper when I was a teen. I did a sixty-page, six-month literature research project on NFP my senior year of college. (Got an A.) I went to introductory sessions for Couple to Couple League and Ovulation Method and felt CCL had the most integrated charting system. I was also impressed with the Los Angeles effectiveness study.[19] With all of the bad things about artificial methods, why would anyone want them?

[19] WADE, ME, MCCARTHY, P, BRAUNSTEIN, GD, ABERNATHY, JR, SUCHINDRAN, CM, HARRIS, GS, et al, A Randomized Prospective Study of the Use-effectiveness of Two methods of Natural Family Planning, Am J Obstet Gynecol, 1981, 141: 368-76.

The difference between NFP and contraception is similar to the difference between euthanasia and allowing someone to die of natural causes. One is an intentional destructive act, but the other is simple nature.

We used this method for three years when we did not have maternity insurance. We had three pregnancies: the first two were achieved on the second month of trying; while the third was a "day sixteen, no mucus due to cold medications, first ovulation post-partum" conception.[20]

However, mine is not necessarily a happy story. I have come to realize it is a common story. America is a multi-cultural, multi-religious country; so often married couples have incompatible values and life goals. Shortly after the birth of our third child, my husband had a vasectomy very much against my consent. We had also just moved, so it was very stressful. He is the kind of guy who always gets what he wants. His goal was probably that he would not ever be responsible for more than three children. Of course it has had a very adverse effect on our marriage, but I do not want this to destroy my family. There are other couples among whom one has been sterilized without the other's consent. Some use NFP for a while and then got sterilized with mutual consent. Others use NFP, but have very strong disagreement over family size.

To complicate this, I have severe dysmenorrhea (painful menstruation). This was treated with sacreal neurectomy. But there were many medical complications and my dysmenorrhea was not totally relieved. Since my husband had a vasectomy, it was strongly recommended that I have a hysterectomy. However, I do not feel like I am finished with having children for some reason.

Periodic abstinence required in NFP is not a big deal. Couples have so much abstinence anyway between health, work, travel, children, and other emotions. It became much easier after my husband's vasectomy since we had so much more distance in our relationship. He had

[20] Editor's note: Regarding this last conception, the return of ovulation after delivery (post-partum) is not predictable. It is indicated by mucus signs which in this case was difficult to observe due to the drying effect of certain cold medications or anti-histamines.

achieved his goal of power and control. Sometimes during phase II both before and after the vasectomy, he would sexually harass me, then ignore me in phase I and phase III.[21] I must have done something wrong somewhere along the line. I believe the pro-life focus should be on abstinence education for the unmarried and economic-social support for the married, so as to increase the odds of a welcomed pregnancy.

Infertility can become a blessing

This couple from California has been married for eight years. He works as a dairy farmer and she as a part-time Registered Nurse. They had been using ecological breast-feeding initially and then Sympto-thermal Method later as an NFP method for the past five years. They have four children including a set of twins.

We would like to tell you how Natural Family Planning has blessed our lives. But, first we think we need to start from the beginning. When we were engaged, we thought it would be a wise decision to postpone pregnancy when we were married. We did hear of NFP from an engaged couple on our Engaged Encounter Weekend. But we knew of no one who actually practiced it. I had irregular cycles and, being a Registered Nurse, doubted the effectiveness of the method. So as a couple we decided to use one of the leading forms of birth control, the pill. It appeared to be less complicated.

We were seven months married when we decided it was time to start our family. To our surprise we were unable to conceive. After being on the pill a little over a year and going off it, I had no cycles. The words *possible side effects* took on a whole different meaning. I was now experiencing a side effect of the pill. Ironically, I began taking my temperature to see if I could conceive a child rather than to postpone a pregnancy-something I had considered too complicated earlier. Six

[21] Editor's note: Phase I and III are the infertile phases before and after ovulation respectively, whereas Phase II is the fertile phase around the time of ovulation.

months of taking my temperature confirmed I was not ovulating. My doctor said I could ovulate tomorrow or never. The thought of not conceiving a child was scary.

The medical way to get my body to ovulate was to take low dose fertility drugs. (With my faith and information I have now, I would have chosen a different route to achieve ovulation.) After taking the fertility drug, we did conceive. Our first child Mary was born, and she was and is a joy. I had intentions of returning to work part-time, but Mary refused to suck from a bottle. I did go to a few *La Leche League* meetings for support. Here I heard of NFP again through a member.

At this point in our lives we were more open to hear more about Natural Family Planning. We attended one class. We learned about NFP and ecological breast-feeding. We decided that I should keep breast-feeding Mary and work minimal hours and leave our fertility to God (which was easy, as we wanted to conceive another child). We conceived again at eleven months postpartum. This happy pregnancy was cut short. At twenty-eight weeks I went into pre-term labor, bed rest followed and a set of twins was delivered at thirty-four weeks. Jenny and Martha were a challenge in our faith. They were small and had to learn to nurse. Jenny was born with a severe physical disability to both lower limbs. With a lot of prayer and support we made it through some tough times. I was able to ecologically breast-feed the twins, and thus extend natural infertility for eleven and a half months. We were very busy and Jenny needed surgery, so that we did not want another child. We dug out *The Art of Natural Family Planning*[22] and read it again. We were sure the Church's teaching against artificial contraception was right, and it was God's will.

I was still nursing our twins and had one long cycle. My experience with interpreting the signs of fertility was minimal. We were banking on another long cycle, and conceived our fourth child. We were upset with ourselves, with God and with NFP. Comments from family, and friends were many and hurtful. We knew how we conceived. We did not follow the conservative rules for beginners who seriously wanted to avoid pregnancy. My main question was, "How could God let us

[22] Editor's note: See Appendix 3

conceive when we were trying to do his will?" Well, grace and peace did come. The tears dried up, and the answer to the question came. It was God's will, not ours. All this time we were praying for our will, assuming it would be God's. We did not realize that God does have total control over all aspects of our lives including our fertility if we allow him, and that his will may not be the same as ours.

Our third pregnancy was good. Labor was difficult. To our surprise we had a healthy baby boy born on the feast day of Our Lady of Guadalupe. He was such a calm and easygoing baby. Jenny learned to walk with her prosthetics that same month. Two great blessings.

Life was even busier now. I breast-fed Andrew, but my cycles did eventually return. I also found out I had stage two cervical dysplasia (abnormal cell growth probable cancer in five to ten years). I now realize that those irregular cycles I had before were due to a nutritional imbalance which was aggravated by the pill as it depletes the body of certain vitamins. My body needed time to heal physically and mentally. We were confused. Tom was doubtful of NFP and our ability to abstain. There was a lot of crying and praying. We found it very difficult at this time to allow God's control over our fertility. Through much prayer, and support from letters from the Couple to Couple League members we decided to try NFP again. This time it was different. We asked the Holy Spirit for wisdom to know the signs God gave my body for the fertile and infertile times, and self-control to abstain as a couple in the fertile time. With God's grace we succeeded.

Now let us go to the beginning, where I mentioned the blessings we have received from practicing NFP. We have four beautiful children and they are blessings from God. At this present moment we are postponing pregnancy, but we know we are doing God's will as we are praying and are open to more children. Artificial contraception and sterilization do not allow God to be there in the marital act. It basically says that you want the pleasure, but not the possible pregnancy that can be a result. "What therefore God has joined together, let no man put asunder." (*Mt.* 19:6) We cannot separate making love and making babies. This is God's natural design. We have realized that God does have control over our lives, even our fertility, when we allow him... And that's a good thing.

As a couple we have grown together physically. We do not take each other for granted, and we have mutual respect for each other. We can talk about anything. We are not bored with each other physically or mentally. Thus our lovemaking is not taken for granted either — each time is special, a total giving of each other, and there is spontaneity (of course, not in the fertile time.) This is the time we learn more about each other's thoughts. We have learned that just holding each other and talking is intimacy, and very rewarding. It is not easy to have self-control sometimes, but this is when we pray to the Holy Spirit for strength. We feel our love for each other is stronger now than on our wedding day.

We have also grown together spiritually. Our faith in God and His Church has grown enormously. We now find time to pray together as a couple and a family. The greatest blessing we feel is knowing that we continue to glorify God even when we make love to each other and this brings great peace.

The little known but amazing advances in NFP

This couple now lives in Nebraska and has use NFP for all the 21 years of their marriage. They have two children aged thirteen and sixteen

I am so happy to tell you about my experience with Natural Family Planning and how it has made a tremendous difference in my life. Currently I am a Registered Nurse who teaches the Creighton Model of Natural Family Planning at Pope Paul VI Institute and it is a very rewarding experience.[23]

[23] In the event you are not familiar with Pope Paul VI Institute, it is a unique combination of many functions that include research and education in human reproduction that was founded in 1985 by Thomas W. Hilgers, M.D., who specializes in Obstetrics and Gynecology. Departments include patient care, reproductive ultrasound center and laboratory, and also the Natural Family Planning Center, which I will focus on. Pope Paul the VI Institute offers accredited educational sessions for the Medical Community who are willing to learn and assist couples with this most important issue. There are also courses offered to help the Clergy understand and speak about NFP. Introductory sessions are held every other Thursday night at the Institute. Then individual follow up sessions are conducted by NFP teachers, who have been trained as Allied Health Professionals. The teachers complete two rigorous Educational Phases that are followed by two supervised practicums. This learning process takes thirteen months and is very thorough. We have a new NFP Teaching Center at the Institute where all instruction takes place. Come and visit us sometime!

My first exposure to NFP was many years ago. I was planning to be married in September of 1976 and was at the physician's office for the necessary exam to receive birth control pills. Like couples of today, I did not know until then about the great and effective option that there was to actually plan our family by using NFP. Nor did I really understand the teachings of our great Roman Catholic Church at this point in my life.

The physician that I visited was Catholic and he highly recommended that I consider using NFP. I was very skeptical, and left the office with the brochure he gave me, disappointed that he had not prescribed pills instead. I seriously doubted that NFP would really work. Looking back, I understand that the "disappointment" was a special blessing.

I followed up on the physician's suggestion, and purchased the book he recommended and basically taught myself the method by reading and applying what I read. Since my husband was Catholic, he agreed to this method and we felt it was successful. It was wonderful not having to rely on chemicals or barriers. Most important, we could enjoy living within the Catholic Church's teaching spelled out so beautifully in *Humanae Vitae*.

Many advances have been made in reproductive health and they are so amazing! Often when I tell others that I am teaching NFP they think I am referring to calendar rhythm — a method that was used many years ago and was very unreliable. I cannot wait to tell them all about how this has changed! The Ovulation Method of Natural Family Planning — Creighton Model — teaches couples how to monitor their combined fertility in a special way that determines the function of the cervix which actually works as a biological valve to inform them of fertility or infertility. Working on this special awareness, the couples mutually share their fertility and use the knowledge to achieve or avoid a pregnancy. It is true family planning, not contraceptive use. It can be used by women in all reproductive categories, including breast feeding, post-partum, pre-menopausal, post pill usage, etc.[24]

[24] HILGERS, T., DAILY, K., HILGERS, S., & PRIBIL, A. *The Ovulation Method of Natural Family Planning: A Standardized, Case Management Approach to Teaching.* Creighton University Natural Family Planning Education and Research Center, 1982.

Today I see a very critical need for more doctors, nurses, and other health professionals to be there for married couples like someone was for me. I'll never forget the doctor that helped me remain contraceptive free and experience the peace that comes from living within the teachings of the Catholic Church. If more of the medical community were willing to refer NFP as the couple's best reproductive option, so many wonderful changes would result. Natural Family Planning's big advantage over artificial contraceptives is that both partners are involved in the use of the method. This enhances communication. Heightened communication cements the marriage bond and results in a special sharing between the couple.

I am so excited to share this great method with interested couples. The method is so easy to learn and use. I hope I have convinced you to come and see for yourself — it's great!

What is Natural Procreative Technology?

This is an excerpt of a talk given by a family doctor from Toronto, Canada. Both she and her husband are physicians. They have been married for seven years and have three sons. In her medical practice, she does not refer for abortions or counsel contraception but promotes NFP, which she also uses in their marriage. She is a Creighton Model Natural Family Planning Medical Consultant.

Good Evening, I am honored to be here tonight to share with you some of my thoughts on the Ovulation Method, Creighton Model of Natural Family Planning. I am not going to be talking about the medical aspect of the method, however, as you might expect from a medical consultant of the method. Instead, I would like to discuss a very important aspect of the Creighton Model, that is, how it responds to the ever pressing threat to human dignity and life in our so-called modern society, as can be seen in the wide spread use of contraceptives and abortion and hence, brings forth the message of *Humanae Vitae*. In short, I would like to explain why I promote the Creighton Model NaProTechnology, not only because of its many medical benefits, but from an ethical point of view as well.

Humanae Vitae, or "Of Human Life," as you know, is the encyclical issued by Pope Paul VI in 1968. There was much anticipation at the time about the Church reversing its position on contraceptive use, after all, a new cultural climate was developing that promotes sexual freedom. With it, however, came the freedom to choose whatever means necessary to avoid pregnancy, and ending any unwanted pregnancy if it occurred, all justifiable in the name of the rights of individual freedom. I recall asking my mother, who is a faithful Catholic about her experience at the time. She was using the calendar Rhythm Method for family planning, but in the span of four years, from 1964 to 1967, she had four children, one each year. So, as you can see, the Rhythm Method did not work. Hence, my mother, like many other Catholics as well as some non-Catholics, hoped and expected the Church to approve the use of contraceptive pills.

However, against much uproar and controversy, the Church "insists that the direct interruption of the generative process already begun must be totally rejected as a legitimate means of regulating the number of children. Similarly there must be a rejection of all acts that attempt to impede procreation, both those chosen as means to an end, and those chosen as ends. This includes acts that precede intercourse, acts that accompany intercourse, and acts that are directed to the natural consequences of intercourse."[25] This is the message of *Humanae Vitae*. Indeed, it is the same position held by the Catholic Church for the past seventeen hundred years.

It is important for us, especially those of us in the field of Natural Family Planning, to understand why the Church remains steadfast in its position in this area. The deeply profound *Humanae Vitae* helps us understands this, and it does so by helping us understand the meaning of love in the Christian marriage. Conjugal love, it explains, is first of all "human," and primarily involves an act of free will whereby spouses strive to persevere through daily joys and sorrows. This love is also "total," whereby the spouses generously share everything with each other without undue reservations. Furthermore, conjugal love is both faithful and exclusive to the end of life. Finally, this love is fruitful, since the whole of love is not contained in the communion of the

[25] *Humanae Vitae*, 14

spouses. Thus, conjugal love requires the spouses to become one in heart and soul and to love unconditionally.[26] The sacrament of marriage is in fact a sign of grace representing the union of Christ and His Church, and Christ's love for his Church is always open to the giving of life. Therefore, the couple's openness to life in procreation is the only appropriate reflection of that love.[27]

Humanae Vitae proclaims that inherent in every act of intercourse are the two inseparable components, union and procreation, that is, love and life.[28] There is simply no natural way where one can experience the sexual act without the possibility of pregnancy. When one uses contraceptives, the unitive and procreative components of the sexual act are separated. As Professor Grondelski, a theologian from St. John's University in New York stated, "When using contraception, I am saying that part of her reality is undesirable, and I intend to destroy it because it interferes with my wish to engage in sexual intercourse. I will express my love for my wife only when she is redesigned according to the image I want her to have at this time. We will make love, but only when she is first outfitted with the proper equipment, be that pharmaceutically (pill), mechanically (IUD) or physically (diaphragm). Ultimately, I do not accept her now as God made her but as I want to remake. This is not love but *use*."[29]

Today's society is excessively concerned with efficiency. Fast food restaurants, microwave ovens, "instant-on" televisions are just a few examples that postponement of gratification can hardly be tolerated. It is no wonder that physicians are also expected to remove every disease, every discomfort from the moment a patient walks into the office. I can certainly relate to the high demands for tranquilizers, diet pills and sleeping pills that seem to offer "quick fixes" for any and all problems. The demand for contraceptives is no different. It is perceived to be something simple, works effectively and devoid of any kind of discomfort. Indeed, it can be obtained by a prescription that takes twenty seconds to write. However, the use of contracep-

[26] *Humanae Vitae*, 9
[27] *Humanae Vitae*, 8
[28] *Humanae Vitae*, 12
[29] GRONDELSKI, JOHN M, *"NFP, Marriage Preparation Counselling and the Clergy" in International Review of NFP*, Spring 1988.

tive pills is associated with a number of side effects, including more serious ones such as thromboembolisms, or blood clots in the leg that can go to the lungs which can be fatal. What is more important, it can act as an abortifacient by preventing the fertilized egg from implanting onto the uterine wall.

Furthermore, the use of contraception to avoid pregnancy has led to a "contraceptive mentality" that perpetuates the diminished tolerance to life, and leads us to believe that intercourse without pregnancy is our right. Larry and Nordis Christenson, a Protestant couple who advocates NFP states, "The contraceptive mentality begins by saying we cannot, will not, must not, shall not, have a baby. If, contrary to our expectation, conception occurs, then abortion could be the next logical step. We have a right to expect that the contraceptive will work, and if it does not, it's not our fault, is it?"[30]

It is frequently asserted that contraception, if made safe and available to all is the most effective remedy against abortion. The Catholic Church is then accused of actually promoting abortion because she continues to teach the moral unlawfulness of contraception. However, the negative values inherent in the contraceptive mentality are such that they in fact strengthen this temptation when an unwanted life is conceived.[31] This can be seen in the case of distributing contraceptives to teenagers in the hope of reducing unwanted pregnancies. A study of teenage sexual practices in the 1970's by the US government and Planned Parenthood, however, revealed that increasing the exposure of teenagers to contraceptive programs actually accelerated the rate of teenage pregnancy and abortion, and that those on the pill are two times more likely to abort than those who were not.[32] In providing teenagers with a program of contraception and thereby encourage them to engage in sexual intercourse, the increase in premarital sex was so great that it surpassed the limits of effectiveness of the birth control and abortion clinics.

[30] CHRISTENSON, LARRY & NORDIS, *"Contraception: Blessing or Blight?", Relevant Issues in NFP,* compiled by THOMAS W. HILGERS, Chapter 17, p.124.

[31] *Evangelium Vitae,* 13.

[32] FORD, JH. & SCHWATZ, M, *Birth Control for Teenagers. Diagram for Disaster, Linacre Quarterly,* Volume 46, Feb. 1979, pp 71-81. *Reprinted in Relevant Issues in NFP.*

So then, what can we do about this depressing state of affairs? I was getting more and more depressed as I was researching this topic. The encyclical *Evangelium Vitae*, or the "Gospel of Life" by Pope John Paul II, provides an even starker picture of our modern world. In addition to the ancient scourges of poverty, hunger, endemic diseases, violence and war, threats to the life of individuals and peoples, especially where life is weak and defenseless, are increasing at an alarmingly fast rate and on a large scale.[33]

This is where the Creighton Model NaProEducation Technology responded to the challenges of *Humanae Vitae*, which appeals to Men of Science, Christian spouses, doctors and health care professionals that through their work, "No true contradictions (will) exist between the divine laws for transmitting life and those for fostering true conjugal love."[34] Most of you are familiar with the Creighton method. It is based upon the couple's own knowledge of their naturally occurring cyclic phases of fertility and infertility, through interpretation of characteristic cervical mucus discharge at certain times of the woman's menstrual cycle. Unlike the calendar Rhythm Method that is highly inaccurate, as discussed earlier, it is 99% effective in avoiding pregnancy when used correctly. It is also very safe, devoid of any side effects and has a very scientific basis.

Is not the Creighton Model just another contraceptive method? A friend of mine asked me once and others may be asking the same question. Is it morally acceptable because it's natural and contraceptives are artificial? This cannot be the reason for in medicine diseases are treated by artificial means with medications and surgery. Clearly that is not morally wrong. In the book *Catholic Sexual Ethics*, the author gives a good explanation: "Some argue that Natural Family Planning and contraception have precisely the same purpose and that therefore they must be morally the same. But this contention involves a fallacy of elementary logic. Two acts — or one act and one deliberate omission — each that has the same purpose need not be morally the same. One can get money to feed one's family by acts of stealing or by honest labor. Though they have exactly the same end, these acts are obvi-

[33] *Evangelium Vitae*, 3
[34] *Humanae Vitae*, 24

ously not morally the same. In practicing NFP a couple adopts a policy to have sexual intercourse at infertile times and to refrain from intercourse at fertile times... Refraining from intercourse is not contraceptive intercourse because it is not intercourse at all."[35]

Another important aspect of the Creighton Model is NaProTechnology. It is a newly emerging science based on research by Dr. Tom Hilgers in the US, where it combines medical, surgical and allied health energies to cooperating with the natural procreative mechanisms of the woman's body.[36] This is an exciting field where through direct input from the woman's charting of her menstrual cycle, various gynecological conditions can be diagnosed and treated. Ovarian cysts, premenstrual syndrome, unusual vaginal bleeding, miscarriage and infertility, are some good examples. I would not go into this any further for it's the subject for another talk. The significance of this development can be seen when we hear this quote from an ardent feminist from Utah who teaches fertility appreciation to her neighbors; she states "We live in a society that does not support women paying attention to their physical and emotional cycles. Much of the medical establishment advance the cult of expert... Doctors are not empowering women to know from inside when that are fertile so they can choose whether to conceive and to use that knowledge as a source of health and creativity."[37] NaProTechnology has become an important part of my medical practice. Especially in the area of infertility, I was able to help a number of couples conceive, but only because of the cooperative nature of the Creighton method where important information was obtained through the woman's charting of her menstrual cycle.

Now, let us go to another issue. Critics of Church policy on contraceptive use commonly ask about "overpopulation." There is a fear of developed nations that if we do not promote and provide contraceptives to the developing countries, there will be a population explosion. Instead of helping the poorer nations achieve access to economic development, the paranoid rich nations have made such access con-

[35] LAWLER, R., BOYLE, J JR. & MAY, WE, *Catholic Sexual Ethics — A Summary, Explanation and Defense, Our Sunday Visitor,* Huntington, Indiana, 1985, p. 168.
[36] HILGERS, T.W., *The Medical Applications of Natural Family Planning: A Contemporary Approach to Women's Health Care,* Pope Paul VI Institute Press, Omaha, Nebraska, 1991.
[37] BAKER, J P, *Conscious Conception, National Catholic Reporter,* April 10, 1992, p. 10.

ditional that they accept their contraceptive programs first. I recall talking to a Creighton Model practitioner-in-training when I was in Omaha, Nebraska learning about the method. She was from Kenya and her anger was almost palpable when she described how the contraceptive pill was forced onto her people. I still remember vividly when she said "they do not want it." In fact, Natural Family Planning is more economical, safer and effective in limiting family size in these countries. When couples in Shanghai, China used the Billings Ovulation Method to avoid pregnancy, a method on which the Creighton Model is based, there is a virtual 100% effective rate.[38] China, as you know, has a strict one-child policy. Another study published in the British Medical Journal where 20,000 East Indian couples were taught Natural Family Planning, it was found to be effective in preventing pregnancies and more than 90% women can be taught to observe signs indicating their natural fertility cycles.[39]

There is no doubt that couples practicing periodic abstinence experience deprivation. However, being aware and tolerant of this deprivation without external coercion, can draw a husband and wife together in a union even stronger than one based on affection alone. Indeed, sexual intercourse does not include only genital intercourse, but encompasses the whole human experience spiritually, physically (not only in the genital sense), intellectually, emotionally and also through effective communication. This is the concept of SPICE with the letters representing each of the areas mentioned, and is an important aspect of the Creighton Model.[40]

The Creighton Model NaProTechnology offers us hope in many ways for a society that seems to promote a "Culture of Death," as Pope Paul II describes it in *Evangelium Vitae.*[41] We must continue the task of promot-

[38] ZHANG, DW & XU, JX, *The Effectiveness of the Ovulation Method Used by 688 Couples in Shanghai,* Shanghai Municipal Family Planning Commission. Presented at the Eleventh Annual Meeting of the American Academy of Natural Family Planning, July 1991, Charleston, West Virginia.

[39] RYDER, REJ, *Natural Family Planning: Effective birth control supported by the Catholic Church, British Medical Journal,* 1993,307: 723-6.

[40] HILGERS, TW, DALY, KD, PREBIL, A.M, HILGERS, SK, *The Ovulation Method of Natural Family Planning: A Standardized, Case Management Approach to Teaching,* Book 1, Creighton University Natural Family Planning Education and Research Center, Omaha, Nebraska, 1982.

[41] *Evangelium Vitae*, 12

ing it as a true method of family planning, in accordance with the dignity of human love and life. I would like to simply close now with this quote from *Humanae Vitae*, "... Truly, just as with all good things outstanding for their nobility and utility, [keeping] the [Divine] law requires strong motivation and much effort from individual Men, from families, and from society. Indeed, this law is not able to be kept without the abundant grace of God, on which the good moral choices of Men depend and from which they get their strength. Moreover, those who consider this matter thoroughly will see that [their] efforts [to keep God's law] increase human dignity and confer benefits on human society."[42]

The truth that sets us free

This couple lives in Ohio. They have been married for five years. They have two children and have used NFP for the five years of their marriage. The husband works as a college mathematics teacher and the wife is a homemaker.

MELISSA: I first heard about Natural Family Planning when I was a senior in high school in 1979. It was a Catholic high school in St. Paul, Minnesota and I was required to take a marriage and family class. A couple came and spoke about NFP. I did not really remember who they were or many of the details about what they said, only that I thought they made a lot of sense. I did not think much about that talk until fourteen years later in 1993 when I met Daniel and we decided to get married. I knew I wanted to learn about NFP. I suggested to Daniel that we take a class in Natural Family Planning to learn the method.

DANIEL: At that time, I knew nothing at all about NFP and very little about the Catholic teaching on sexuality, despite the fact that I was an adult covert to Catholicism for nearly 11 years. I came to faith in Jesus and was baptized in a Southern Baptist church at age thirteen. I became Catholic at age twenty-two while in the US Navy. This is not the place to retell that story, but it might be important to try to explain how it is that I had been Catholic so long without knowing about my Church's teaching on such an important matter.

[42] *Humanae Vitae*, 20

The fault was mostly my own; it was a lack of faith. To be sure, the priest who had given me instructions was not very accurate in presenting the Church's teaching. As best as I can recall, the view he presented was very similar to what I would later learn was that of the majority of the Papal Birth Control Commission. That really was not excusable since it was 1982 and *Humanae Vitae* had long since been released. Still, I was fairly sure that the actual position of the Church was more strongly against contraception than that priest had admitted. The trouble was that I was afraid to find out what that position was. Please understand that I was not at all afraid that the Catholic Church might be right (and that I would therefore never be able to use contraceptives). Quite to the contrary, I was afraid that the Church would be clearly wrong. That would most likely mean the end of my faith.

While there were several reasons that I became Catholic (attraction to liturgical worship, the example of friends who were Catholic, etc.), The most important, I think, was that I could no longer believe in "private interpretation of Scripture." (If you need a further explanation, I could provide one of course, but it would take more than a few words.) The Catholic Church provided me with the only way out. I could keep my faith in Jesus Christ because, in His Church, he had provided the solution to the problems of private interpretation that were torturing me. I knew, too, that the Catholic Church seemed to be right on at least some issues (such as giving an interpretation of the sixth chapter of St. John's Gospel that would make any sense). So, as best as I remember, I became Catholic because it offered the only reasonable alternative to no faith at all.

Yet, I knew that if the Magisterium taught error in even one instance, then the whole of Catholic theology collapsed too. And I feared very much that I would discover that Church teaching on contraception was the big joke that most of my friends thought it was. Rather than face my fears, I remained ignorant. I also remained a rather lukewarm Catholic.

I would like to mention that contraception was not the only issue that scared me. I was also scared about the basis for baptism of infants, the veneration of saints, and Mary's perpetual virginity, just to name a few. Slowly, God worked to help me discover that, in case after case, the Catholic Church was *right* after all! With every such discovery, my faith was made stronger. I even began to consider religious life. However, I still knew practically nothing about the Church's teaching on marriage and sexuality. In hindsight, it may have been my last and biggest intellectual obstacle to a full embrace of the faith. Had I actually become a monk, I wonder when I would have gotten the courage to confront my fear of this issue. Perhaps that is "the reason" why God did not call me to serve him in the monastery, if one can speak in this way.

In any case, I had fairly well discerned that my vocation was not to be a religious when, in 1993, I met Melissa. My love for her was all it took to give me the courage to "face my fear" and take a class in NFP. Of course, once again, my fears were groundless. Not only was the Church not wrong about this, she was so overwhelmingly, obviously *right* — I almost could not believe what I was learning. Discovering that *all* Christian denominations rejected contraception until about 1930 (a fact that is freely admitted by those on all sides of this issue) was a real bombshell for me. Also, I began to discover that all of the moral teachings of the Church concerning sexuality, most of which I already accepted, really began to make sense for the first time. I realized *why* sex was wrong outside of marriage, *why* homosexuals could not simply be allowed to marry, and so forth.

Also, I was relieved to discover the solid scientific basis for Natural Family Planning. I was never really convinced that the "overpopulation scare" was anything other than scientific fraud. However, I was glad to know that there were morally acceptable and medically reliable ways to limit the number of births in whatever instances it might be prudent to do so. I did not (and do not) believe that God simply wants all couples to have as many children as possible. With NFP as an option, one can prudently limit one's family size, and possibly advise others to do the same, without demanding supernatural or heroic virtue of anyone.

MELISSA: Fortunately, we cannot make any fair comparison of NFP to contraception in marriage, but we do believe that practicing NFP is good for marriage. When we got married in December 1993, we were seeking pregnancy as soon as possible. We had several months of experience in charting and interpreting signs of fertility before conceiving in August 1994. Therefore we had no actual experience with the use of NFP to postpone pregnancy until after Emily was born in May of 1995. Then, we had to practice complete abstinence for several months. Breast-feeding had several effects. For one thing, the signs of fertility, mucus and temperature, were completely different and unpredictable. The other effect was that I was completely exhausted, both physically and emotionally. I had no desire for (and not a little fear of) another pregnancy any time soon. And although I was exclusively breast-feeding, I lacked confidence in it as a method of birth control. The only option, then, was abstinence.

Far from being a bad experience, I think this period of abstinence was one of the most valuable experiences of our marriage. For one thing, we found out that we really did believe in the Church's teachings, even when they were hard to follow. For another, we learned not to take sexual intimacy, even in marriage, for granted. I think I also got a lot of confidence in my husband's sexual self-control. Based on comments I have heard from friends, I am not sure that all women have the confidence that their husbands can "do without." But does not a wife need that confidence?

DANIEL: Following that period of complete abstinence was a period of periodic abstinence when fertility cycles finally returned. Perhaps it is just a matter of personal taste, but I believe this "natural rhythm" of abstinence followed by sexual intimacy is precisely the way to keep a sort of "honeymoon excitement" in a marriage. I really like it.

MELISSA: We both have complete confidence in the effectiveness of Natural Family Planning. While we have absolutely no scientific basis for saying this, we both believe that if a woman knows her fertility signs well enough, and if a little extra abstinence is acceptable, NFP is virtually 100% effective. And if we ever did have an unplanned pregnancy, I'll bet we would know "why?" Somehow, I think that would make the "surprise" much easier to deal with. In contrast, we have two different friends who have each gotten pregnant while taking the pill without ever missing a single day (or so they say). And neither of them has the slightest idea of what "went wrong." By the way, one of those friends, a Protestant, is now using NFP and giving Janet Smith's tapes to all her friends.

I do not want to be treated as a toy

This couple from Maryland has been married for two years. They have been using NFP for these two years and do not have any children as yet.

I live near Washington, DC in Maryland and have been married for almost two years. I began charting my cycle six months before that. My twin sister and I are the youngest of nine children. My parents did not attempt to use any kind of contraception, and did not know about NFP. In fact their initial response to us using it was skepticism. They did not believe that it worked. And they did not believe that two people who were in love and married could choose to abstain. In any case, these objections are not unreasonable. I must say that since my husband and I chose to wait until he was finished with his Ph.D., It has not always been easy to wait until days of infertility.

Practicing Natural Family Planning has become easier with time, and we are now hoping to conceive. In watching friends and colleagues who have kids when they did not plan to have them, or those who long for children and are unable to conceive, I am continually reminded that the birth of a child is first of all, a gift, and not something entirely in our hands. Otherwise, it is too easy to use NFP as another form of birth control.

There are two immediate benefits from using Natural Family Planning. First, I see the sad results of using artificial contraceptives, especially in my colleagues. It is a lie which reduces the woman to a toy. This creates resentment and even bitterness against their boyfriend or husband. As a result, there is a scorn for motherhood in all its aspects where children are only perceived as major inconveniences. The second benefit of NFP is that I am much more in tune with my body, and that I can communicate this to my husband.

Having said this, I must say that NFP does ask for a certain amount of sacrifice which would be unreasonable for me to take on without the help of the Church. In other words, I know that it is better for me not to drink coffee, but I enjoy it, and so I continue. I know it is better for me not to cuss, but it has become a habit, and so I continue it even if I want to stop. The reasons of "being natural" and "doing the right thing" are not enough. The Church has a very concrete face for me in the movement "Communion and Liberation." Watching my friends suffer the consequences of using artificial contraceptives, I am constantly reminded of the value of following the Church in all its particulars.

How to overcome the contraceptive mentality

This couple from Nebraska has been married for thirty-five years and they have been using NFP for twenty-eight years. Other than being a wife and mother of four, she is a professional freelance writer and a paraprofessional for disabled children. She also volunteers at a crisis pregnancy center which she was a past director, and teaches NFP. The husband works as a high school teacher.

We learned about NFP from a marriage preparation course *Cana Is Forever.* At that time, NFP was simple and our instruction may have filled one whole paragraph, but it worked quite well for us. We practiced NFP because that is what the Church taught.

Natural Family Planning differs from contraception because it does not harm the mother or the child. Contraception on the other hand stands between God and life. This is understandable when you consider that the birth control pill alone has more than seventy possible side-effects for mother and child. Granted, some medicines have more side effects than the pill, but the pill in contrast is for healthy, not unhealthy people. The pill does not treat diseases. Pregnancy is not a disease. When we are sick, we have a legitimate reason to use medicine until the underlying disease vanishes. Those who take the pill for the "disease of pregnancy" harm their bodies in the process. Furthermore, NFP differs from contraception because some forms of unnatural birth control such as the pill, Norplant, Depo-Provera, and the IUD are abortifacient.[43] We have several generations of parents that

[43] Editor's note: See note 6 for details.

either do not know these grave facts or do not care. Our Lord must be very discontented when we abuse our bodies and those of our children in these ways.

The Rhythm Method worked well for us, but the new Sympto-thermal Method that we later used was more accurate. In essence, we had three unplanned pregnancies, but not because of a method failure. We just became lax when it seemed we might want another child. Our love, not the pill, determined when we should have another child. We have four children. We consider all of them gifts from God.

Too many mothers with unplanned pregnancies are using chemical birth control at the time of conception. The pill, or whatever they used is not foolproof. God chooses to give these mothers gifts of new life, too. However, we worry about all the health effects from using the chemicals when pregnancy occurs. We wonder, too, about the spiritual deprivation of not following God's will — first they contracept, and then they abort.

The periodic abstinence, when using NFP, is an advantage rather than a disadvantage to married couples. There is a honeymoon and wedding every month. God knew what he was doing when he created us. If statistics show that contracepting couples have marital relations four to seven times per month, then NFP users surely have a better track record than that! NFP couples stay together at the rate of 95% or better. Is not that enough proof that ten or twelve days of abstinence per month works?

The population explosion is a myth. The entire population on this planet could hold hands around the coast of the British Isles.[44] Does that sound like overpopulation? Of course not. In our thinking, the population myth was devised by those who had a great deal of money to profit from selling birth control and abortion. These "experts" do not operate on a high spiritual level; even though their environmental motives mistakenly sound good.

[44] Editor's note: This is a calculation to show that the world has a lot more space to hold the 6 billion inhabitants. Another similar calculation is that the whole population of the world can stand in an area of 143 square miles, which is 20% of the city Jacksonville, Florida. For a complete treatment of the subject of population read *Handbook on Population,* ROBERT L SASSONE, American Life League, Inc, 1998, 6th ed.

I, Mary, now teach NFP. I wish I had started many years earlier. The world fumes in turmoil because of a contraceptive mentality. This twisted way of thinking has led to immorality, teen pregnancy, abortion, lack of full-time mothers, absent fathers, divorce, abuse, government solutions, and more. Paul VI predicted much of this back in 1968 when he gave us *Humanae Vitae*. I wonder if I could have prevented a small amount of disharmony if I had started teaching NFP sooner.

The method worked for us

This is a testimony from California. They have been married for fifteen years with one daughter, age nine. They have used NFP method approximately twelve years.

I am a wife, married close to fifteen years. I am now in the menopause and no longer need the Natural Family Planning method although I have been very happy with it. I believe I learned about NFP in marriage preparation classes. Since I have used it, I found that it was more fail-safe than is generally believed. A lot of people think of it only as the Rhythm Method and Russian roulette. NFP is just abstinence at the fertile time, and it has an easy, practical method of determining the fertile times. For it to be effective, care must be taken to really watch the signs.

Natural Family Planning worked beautifully in my case. I got pregnant instantly when we decided to "pull the plug" as we joke about it. We watched for the signs of maximal fertility, had sex at that time on a very nice vacation in Hawaii, and came back from the trip with my daughter on the way.

I did not get pregnant when I was trying not to. Once, when we were undecided about having a child earlier in our marriage and decided not to try hard either way, I got pregnant after some months but had a miscarriage. This was actually a good thing because we felt it was not the right time for us to have a child. Although I had the miscarriage, I was also willing to accept the will of the Lord if the pregnancy had come to term.

I was fine with the need for periodic abstinence in the NFP method. I do not think abstinence was an obstacle to intimacy or unnatural. Throughout history, couples have been separated for long times through business, war, or perhaps hunting for food in primitive times, and certainly through death. The natural human state is to have separations at times, to be without a partner. When couples then get back together, it can be especially happy after abstinence. Relations are less likely to become a humdrum routine. My husband was less enthusiastic. He would have liked no time of abstinence and saw no need for this method, even though he agreed that it was an effective one.

Another advantage of using NFP is that it is natural and healthy. I never had a yeast infection or any other "female troubles." I attribute my good health to not interfering with my body with any chemicals as I have never used artificial contraception, not even the condom.

Before engaging in sex, more people should try to think of the ultimate consequences: a child. It is a *major* step and a *giant* consequence. Hollywood only emphasizes the fun and glory of sex but not the tremendous consequences. It is really playing with fire. If people would think before they act, there would be fewer unexpected pregnancies and thus the need for abortion. They would be better stewards of the earth.

The deeper meaning of human sexuality

This couple from Ontario, Canada has been married for more than three years and they have used NFP since their marriage. At the time when this was written, they were expecting the arrival of their first child.

We cannot remember how or when we first learned of Natural Family Planning, but certainly, we learned of it before we ever met and started dating. I may have learned of it from a married couple I met when I was a university undergraduate — a wonderful Catholic couple I admired very much. We never shared the popular misconception that

NFP is haphazard or ineffective, but we did lack specific information about the female fertility cycle.

I never realized the importance of good cervical mucus for conception. Indeed, I do not think the basic health classes I had in public schools ever mentioned the existence of cervical mucus but only that an egg and a sperm were present. I also thought I would have to check about six different things every day in order to determine my fertility, when in fact I only need to check one thing — the color, stretchability and sensation of my cervical mucus.

My husband thought that the individual female cycles were more uniform than they really are, and was surprised that my periods are so long or that I have longer than a 28-day cycle. He also did not understand female mood swings and felt frustrated at his inability to predict them. Charting my fertility helped him to see when I might not be at my best, so that he could be more patient and avoid important discussions at those times.

Obviously, NFP meets the objective moral criteria for regulation of births as explained by the Catholic Church, while contraception does not. These are clear enough in *Humanae Vitae* and the *Catechism of the Catholic Church*, among other writings.

Personally, I see contraception as the attempt to find a "No Thought, No Action, No Effort" solution to the possible problems of fertility and family planning. Contraceptive users live in ignorance of the natural, healthy workings of the body as well as the deeper meanings of nature, sexuality, and procreation. They do not practice discipline to influence whether or not they will conceive. Rather, they attempt to render procreation impossible with little or no effort by external means be they pills, implants, or surgery. They think they can pick a piece of artificial junk and never have to think or worry about the situation again. But the many negative personal and social consequences of contraception should show us all that this practice does not hold up under the weight of reflection and experience.

Similarly, I feel that couples who reject NFP as well as rejecting contraception should also be careful of this "No Thought, No Action, No Effort" mentality. I realize that they are not like couples who use immoral birth control methods. When they are not actively engaged in a behavior that requires daily discipline and reflection, they may not have fully reflected upon their duties to God, to each other in their marriage, to their children or family, and to their society. They, especially the wives, may never know how wonderfully made they are thanks to God because they lack information which could be important for protecting their fertility, their unborn children, and their general gynecological health. Also, they may not have reflected deeply on the sexual aspect of their marriage. In short, when it comes to sex and procreation, they may find it easier to just have sex whenever they feel like it without having to reflect and decide about it every day.

Again, I respect the personal decisions of these couples. Many of them are faithful, practicing Catholics who feel they are showing trust in God by "letting him decide how many children they should have." However, the decision to have sex whenever they feel so inclined is, in itself, also a family planning decision. It should be one which should stem from reflection, and not from laziness or a desire to take the easiest way. After all, our lives, health, livelihoods and material possessions are dependent on God every moment. Accidents, upsets, and disasters can and do happen at any time; he who pretends otherwise is kidding himself. We show trust and hope in God every day that we live. But I thought I should say that couples who reject NFP might really be missing out on something very good for themselves, their marriage, and their relationship with God.

NFP does work, and I would say it was 100% effective for us. When we were married, for various reasons we felt we should delay the beginning of our family. We did not conceive any children in the two and a half years of using NFP. Then, when it was time to start a family, we conceived a baby in the second month we tried. We knew exactly when I ovulated, and God was promptly generous to us in our obvious request for a baby.

Natural Family Planning has taught me that fertility and sexuality are more complex than I had originally thought. It helped me to experience firsthand the truth and importance of *Humanae Vitae*, which describes benefits far beyond the mere spacing of children. To begin with, NFP information provides for many medical benefits, of which the general public seems unaware. I also learned the value of understanding, admiring, and cooperating with God's natural order, especially that of the female fertility cycle. And by continuing to develop chastity, which my husband and I practiced before marriage, I learned the truth that it can become the root of many other virtues. I always thought that will power is what makes a marriage successful and permanent. *Humanae Vitae* calls this quality "self-mastery" and teaches us that the control of our sexual drives is one of the best places to start developing this virtue which makes a marriage last.

In general, I think that periodic abstinence seems to sound less ideal to my husband than to me. However, he does not seem to regard it as a great trial or major annoyance. I think that he was strong and patient enough to defer sex until he married at twenty-five, and was then very much looking forward to having sex. He seems ready to have sex more often. However, he already had character enough to practice NFP, so I cannot say it was a serious strain. Having a regard for his feelings, I always let him know that if he really wanted to have intercourse, even if I was fertile and we were supposedly not starting our family yet, I was willing to have intercourse and I felt we could do our best with the baby. He might think about it for a minute then, but he never took me up on this offer.

Now that we have started our family (I'm pregnant with our first child), I can look back and say that avoiding or achieving pregnancy did not make much difference in our sex lives. We had intercourse with the same frequency in both seasons of our marriage. That suggests to me that NFP was not the deciding factor, but that we had struck a balance, or developed a pattern, which accounted for our feelings, as well as distractions like work, fatigue, or illness, without specific regard to family planning goals.

Personally, I think that periodic abstinence helped me a great deal in terms of marital satisfaction. After protecting my virginity until marriage at twenty-five, I realized that chastity had become an important part of my identity and self-esteem; I was a little worried about losing this, losing part of myself as I knew myself, when I got married. I knew that I would have to develop a new sense of self and did not have a good idea how I would do this. I felt that NFP let me adjust to married life a bit more gradually, since I did not have to shift from virginity to some kind of orgy! My husband and I maintained a kind of chastity appropriate to our new state of life. Also, I often felt a little sore, physically, when I first became sexually active, and I was glad to have some days to let my body recover. But I never felt that I had to displease my husband in order to get a break. Moreover, I was susceptible to feelings of being unloved, and of being used as an object, when my husband seemed less interested in the hand holding, hugging, and kissing which had been part of our courtship. I understood that he now had something more "interesting" in intercourse, but I valued love indications outside of sex to show that I was still a person to him and still loved. NFP helped us keep a balance.

I would like to see more exploration of NFP in terms of a spiritual good. Pope John Paul II writes of the development of virtue, especially in marriage, as a process (see *Familiaris Consortio*, 32-35). And NFP is also a process, since couples practicing it may not fully appreciate what it is and what it has to offer until they experience it and reflect on the experience. As Catholics, we appreciate the use of ritual to deepen our spiritual life, and NFP serves as a kind of ritual too, serving the sacrament of marriage. I would like to see theologians and experts write more on NFP in this sense — as a possible devotional practice which helps us more deeply understand creation and the relationship of God to man, married couples, and families. After all, there are many different sorts of devotions and spiritual expressions encouraged by the Church, such as almsgiving or devotion to saints, which are not specifically required but which add much to spiritual life. Even if a couple begins with a "less than ideal" understanding of the use of NFP, they have still begun a process of cooperating with God's natural order and with each other, and improving their health (in contrast with contraceptive measures). One decent action can lead to another and then another. In practicing NFP, and acquiring good habits (of respect for the body and of marital abstinence), then, I think we improve ourselves as people. And it may do couples more good than they realize, not simply because of the influence of a good NFP instructor, but because God has a chance to work on them as well.

Getting pregnant will be dangerous for my health

This testimony comes from a couple from Illinois. The wife is a schoolteacher and the husband a farmer. They have used Natural Family Planning for more than nineteen years and have two children ages sixteen and nineteen.

We were married in 1975. Our *Pre-Cana* marriage preparation classes spent the better part of an afternoon presenting various contraceptive methods of birth control (in a manner mostly contradicting Church teaching). Toward the end of the session, the existence of natural methods of family planning was "acknowledged."

Being from strong Catholic families, we opted to follow Church teachings and rely on calendar rhythm. Besides, we wanted children and did not view them as a "plague." We did have a fairly important reason to delay pregnancy as I, Irene, needed to teach for two years after graduation or pay back my scholarship in full... God was good to us in this matter, and we conceived on our first attempt two years later.

In 1978, after a difficult delivery, our doctor informed us that we were not to conceive again for two years due to my health. He wanted to know what would we do to accomplish this. Guidance from pastors varied widely. We decided to confide in the priest who celebrated our wedding. But his answer, "You have a tough one!" Was really not an answer at all. Then our church bulletin announced Natural Family Planning classes sixty miles away. We went to prove to ourselves that NFP would not work, salve our consciences and choose contraceptives for medical reasons. We wonder how many others have not been as fortunate as we were in this situation, as just the opposite happened. Looking back, we probably were reacting to the pressure we were under as artificial contraception was still against our principles.

Our second pregnancy was much more difficult than our first one. I had gallstones and hypoglycemia. The uterus contained too much fluid, a sign of possible kidney problems in the baby. One of my kidneys was enlarged, too. During this second C-section delivery my appendix was "hot" and was removed. Three months later my gallbladder was removed. Once again we had serious reasons to avoid pregnancy but we did not doubt our choice of NFP.

In 1986 we put our trust in God to try for a daughter. Yes, we conceived, but six weeks later we experienced trouble. Our NFP charts were the only reason I had even seen a doctor because it was the first time I felt fine at the onset of pregnancy. A physical exam for pregnancy was negative, but the blood tests (and charts) were positive. Something was wrong. I had an ectopic[45] pregnancy. We lost our third child, not understanding the Lord's timing.

Our faith was put to the test. We often asked why we could not have more children. Our basketball team had only two members (our two sons), but we felt that perhaps God was calling us to be NFP teachers.

Since 1991 we have been sharing our NFP knowledge and experiences with others as a Couple to Couple League teaching couple. NFP forces couples to communicate on a vital ingredient of their marriage. As a result, communication is strengthened in general. Periodic abstinence protects the marriage from boredom — "abstinence" makes the heart grow fonder. Mutual respect is attained. With NFP, couples work together on family planning, whereas with contraceptives the "burden" often rests with one spouse. Communication suffers and mutual respect is lost.

Twenty years later we can say NFP has been a major blessing in our marriage. It has become a way of life. The rewards far outweigh the difficulties. When we started out in 1975, the Church was in turmoil on the issue of birth control. Today in many ways it still is. Yet today the Church and especially our current pontiff, Pope John Paul II, speak more definitively and thoroughly on this topic. In 1975, we remained faithful to Church teaching by the grace of God and the strength of our upbringing and beliefs. At that time, we did not understand the Church's teaching, but we accepted it. Since then, we have come to understand as well as accept it. Perhaps, as has been our experience, the Lord has his own schedule.

Will there be difficult moments with NFP? Yes, but difficulty is not necessarily bad. To quote our doctor as a storm front approached while we awaited the birth of our *three-week overdue* first child, "Storms bring great things."

[45] Ectopic pregnancies are pregnancies that did not take place in the womb (uterus) but somewhere else, normally in the fallopian tubes. They are also called tubal pregnancy. These pregnancies will not come to term and are dangerous for the mother's health from internal bleeding. Surgical treatment is necessary.

Abstinence is for real men and real women

Dr. John Hillabrand was one of the pioneers of natural methods of family planning back in the 1930's. When Dr. Hillabrand attended a meeting in Kansas City years ago, he was so impressed with a talk a woman gave that he asked her to write it. The following is what she wrote. The original writer could not be traced and Dr. Hillabrand has passed away.

Dear Dr. Hillabrand,

It is hard for me to put down on paper exactly what I felt and said that night in Kansas City. I can tell you that I meant every word of it. For the sake of your couples I will try to write it all down. I think the best advice I could give to anyone giving a talk on periodic abstinence using the Basal Temperature Technique would be to look deeply into their own attitude toward it. Look long and hard and see how they really feel toward it. It also helps, as I have done, to observe closely, couples who use contraceptives and listen to what they say and do not say. In a sense put their marriage against yours and see how it measures up. I do not know about your couples but contraceptive marriages against ours come out a poor second. Here are couples who have all the wonders of modern science, all the pills, jellies, coils, etc. And yet very little sexual maturity and very little concept of human love. I do not say that in judgment but only out of great sadness for them.

I feel that if you start out a marriage with unlimited and undisciplined intercourse, you will never know the tenderness of waiting patiently or impatiently for it. Even from impatience you can learn a great deal about yourself and your husband. You learn to be tender, to be considerate, in short you learn to love this man you have decided to live with the rest of your life. You discover things about him you otherwise never would. In a way, abstinence and its acceptance become a test and thus an ultimate proof of your love. You may fall and fall many times, but from each time you will learn-to give a little more, to love a little more.

One thing I think most women will get out of it is a great respect for their husbands and that certainly cannot hurt these days. When a woman respects her husband, she will soon grow to adore him. When he sees the respect in her attitude, he can only see to strive harder to please her. Their love can only grow and grow in this type of atmosphere despite the adversity and trials of daily living. In a way it is like having the most wonderful secret in the world.

If this sounds like a saccharin existence, it is not. You fight, you bicker, you nag, and you make up. You sacrifice. You smile when you do not feel like it. You do some crying, too. But look what you have — a good man's deep and abiding love and a good woman's deep and abiding love and surrender. It is not just our marriage I'm speaking of but countless other couples we have met and talked to.

We would never have known each other in this way if we had not been abstaining at one time or another. Abstinence gives you a time for pause. You look more deeply at this man you have married. You now have an opportunity to see beyond his body and your own. Perhaps this is where we get a glimpse of the soul.

So, I guess this, in essence, is why we're blessed and why I feel sorry for people who will never know this. To me they are half-alive. The mercy is that they are not aware of it or they could never stand living the way they are. I know that I would never trade places with them for anything in the world. They have sexual intercourse as often as they want, but little sexuality. The men are not men and the women will never know what it means to be a real woman, because only a real man can lead a woman to the realization of herself.

It is something really wonderful, when the day after the safe period ends, your husband hugs and kisses you and you realize "he loves me for myself and not just for my body." How can you ever feel this way if you use contraceptives? It is a feeling no woman should miss experiencing. Abstinence can be an enriching experience rather than a misfortune.

A doctor's testimony — My conscience in clear

This testimony comes from a physician in Minnesota.

For me it really began with marriage and the personal decision regarding how we would responsibly plan our family. As we talked with my fiancé's parents in 1981, they shared their knowledge and experience, both the Church's teaching and their experience working with engaged couples in the St. Paul Minneapolis diocese. And as any good medical student would do, I researched the Church's writings, the theological literature, and the medical literature. It became clear to me that our Church was teaching throughout the ages including the present days, the revealed knowledge of God. He made us in his image and likeness. To disregard the truth he has given us about ourselves would only lead us down paths away from God and from his desires for our life and works in this world.

After making this decision in my married life, I knew I would need to remain consistent in my medical practice. I therefore researched how I could incorporate this into my vocation and chose to enter into the practitioner and medical consultant programs at Creighton University under the direction of Dr. Tom Hilgers in 1982. Those are now taught through the American Academy of Natural Family Planning (AANFP).

In 1983-86 I went through a residency in Family Practice in Minneapolis through the University of Minnesota. During that period I submitted a proposal to the hospital which resulted in the moving of the Twin Cities Natural Family Planning Center to the hospital campus. I thus had access to practitioner services for my patients, and also served as the medical director.

I then went into practice in 1986 and joined another physician who also followed the Church's teaching in moral matters. I eventually hired an NFP practitioner to teach in my clinic, and also helped Twin Cities NFP locate practitioners in other clinics to provide on site services to patients. This also made it easier for patients to utilize their insurance for payment coverage. I have remained peripherally active in the AANFP and have served on the diocesan NFP board and Ethics committee.

Throughout my changing career I have never prescribed contraceptives for family planning purposes. The Lord has blessed me greatly through my decisions to follow his Word as revealed through the Roman Catholic Church. I have been given wonderful patients, the chance to witness and help those having difficulty with decisions in the area of sexuality, and the ability to live with a clear conscience that I am following his will for me as his son. To disregard God's moral truths leads to consequences far greater than when we disobey his scientific truths; the results are just a little slower in their appearance.

The difficulties and benefits of abstinence

This is a testimony that comes from Michigan. The couple has use NFP for twenty years. They have been married for 23 years and have 3 children. The husband works in advertising and the wife is a homemaker.

During my last semester Kendall School of Design in 1974, just turning twenty-two, I had been practicing anew my Catholic faith for about a year. I would walk to class early in the morning and pray the rosary. In my petitions, I remember requesting to meet a girl that I could share my faith and life with. Six weeks before graduation, I was introduced to Nancy, a student in Illustration. I called to ask her out to a movie. I did not have a car so we walked. The walk gave us time to talk and share our backgrounds. I knew in my heart, after that first date, she was the one to marry. We dated for six months and then became engaged for six months. At this time we made the decision to stay chaste. It was, to say the least, no small challenge. Through the grace of God we refrained from the sexual embrace until our wedding day. We were going to wait a couple of years before having children so that we would "get to know each other."

Our honeymoon was a trip to Montreal, Canada. I thought Nancy would go on the pill. She wanted to try "Rhythm." Her girlfriend had told her to watch out for day 14. Nancy did not have regular cycles and so our first son John was born nine months to the day of our wedding. We got to "know each other" very quickly. We were actually thrilled with the arrival of our son. He was the first grandchild on both sides. We thought would we give Rhythm another try and Jacob was born eighteen months after John. I think Jacob might have come sooner if Nancy were not breastfeeding our firstborn. Anyway we were thrilled once again.

We had always wanted a family but we wanted some space in between pregnancies. Nancy was happy but a little overwhelmed those first couple of years. While reading Sheila Kippley's book, *Breastfeeding and Natural Child Spacing,* she came across a reference about the Sympto-thermal Method of family planning from the Couple to Couple League. Nancy requested and received information on this method and told me there would be times of abstinence. I love my wife and told her, "I'll be strong — just tell me when." I was still burdening Nancy with the responsibility of family size and fertility awareness. At first she studied on her own but later signed up for a class by a certified teaching couple. After taking the classes once a month for four months (two hours per session), I came to realize that we needed to share this responsibility of family planning. My involvement was to give Nancy the thermometer each morning at the same time and then chart the temperature. Also, I began to take the responsibility of interpreting the time of infertility. This took a lot of the burden of getting pregnant off Nancy. It was very easy to observe the fertile and infertile phases. God designed the woman's body perfectly.

Practicing abstinence during the fertile time, to postpone pregnancy, became an opportunity to direct our energies in the service of others. This challenged us to show our love in other positive ways other than the sexual embrace. We learned how to offer up this time of abstinence, a small sacrifice, for the engaged, our priest and people struggling with chastity.

Our daughter Joanne was born five years after Jacob. We came to notice over the years that the times of abstinence created a courtship/honeymoon relationship each month. We looked forward to the times of renewing our marriage covenant. Abstinence has kept the spark alive in our marriage. Also, abstinence has taught us self-control, helping us to master our sexual urges in all its forms. When there are difficult times of temptation we ask God and the Blessed Virgin Mary for help. The practice of self-control in our sexuality has extended into other areas of daily living such as moderation in eating, drinking and television. It has helped in developing those virtues we need in raising and forming our children into Christian adults.

Over the years, the greatest gift has been the moral consistency with our children. We have asked them to remain sexually pure and chaste until marriage. We know that this is possible because of our own lives. This has not been without challenge, but we have been able to talk about sexuality more openly with them, answering to many of today's arguments in defense of God's ways. John is now serving in the navy. He practices his Catholic faith and looks forward to marriage and family someday. Jacob is a religious brother with the Legionaries of Christ. Joanne, an active teenager, has promised (and was given a gold ring to remind herself) to keep chaste until marriage. However, as I said before, none of these has been without its trials.

We continue to acknowledge and practice the truth of Christ's teaching in sexuality, and we also embrace the Church and all her teachings. The pope is the Vicar of Christ among us upholding and teaching God's truths. The world is forever bombarding us with sexual temptations. Natural Family Planning has been a gift from God that has helped us in this struggle. It has added so much more to our marriage than just a method of spacing children. In the teaching of CCL, which includes a theology of the body consistent with Catholic doctrine, we have gained a whole new appreciation of procreation and the union of husband and wife.

Sex is a lifelong project

"This testimony arrived from a Puerto Rican couple who have been married and used NFP for six years. They have a three-year-old child and the husband works in claim adjustment".

WIFE: I knew that artificial methods were not for us from my values and psychological, physical and emotional health. I discussed this with my boyfriend and he agreed. Just as we decided to get married, our decision was made to not use anything other than a natural method. The question was which one to choose — calendar rhythm or ovulation. I wanted something more complete and I was pretty worried. But God led us to the pre-marriage workshop in *Casa Manresa* where we found the method we wanted to use, the Sympto-thermal Method. Our lives changed forever and for good with the telephone number of a teaching couple.

HUSBAND: Natural methods are different from contraception because they are healthy and good for the growth of a couple's relationship. They do not affect the moral values that our parents have transmitted to us about God's teachings. Many couples go through marriage just thinking of sex because society presents it in an erroneous manner. It is not until we get married that we recognize that sex is a lifelong project. It requires understanding and communication between each other. We have known couples who divorced the first night of the honeymoon because "lovemaking" was not as they imagined. Many couples get married ignoring this fact.

WIFE: I thank God for my husband and this method. He's so understanding and communicative. We usually talk a lot on the days we practice abstinence and that helps us grow as a couple. We think that in our case the natural planning has been a blessing to us, because we have not allowed sex to be a priority in our lives, like other couples we know that have been unsuccessful in their marriage. In our honeymoon, we could not have intercourse because we wanted to postpone. My cycle was anovulatory[46] and so we had to wait a month until our marriage was consummated. We understood, since the beginning, that sex is not for a moment but it is forever.

HUSBAND: We think God has different plans for every couple. Our first baby was unplanned, but God sent a lot of messages that made us sure it was the right time for a baby to come.

WIFE: I knew I ovulated and was very sure I became pregnant. Two weeks later, I went to a checkup with my doctor and he reassured I

[46] Editor's note: Anovulatory cycles are menstrual cycles where there are no ovulations. Since all NFP methods determine if a woman is fertile or not based on the presence of signs of ovulation, in anovulatory cycles one cannot accurately predict the phases of fertility. See Appendix 1 for further explanation.

was pregnant. It was God's plan, not ours. This made us believe more in the natural method. It's so great to know what's happening in my body. We have been using the method for six years and are now certified as a teaching couple for Couple to Couple League.

Our relationship grew in using NFP

Now living in Quebec, Canada, this couple has been married for nine years and has one child with two years of age. They have been using Natural Family Planning to help them achieve pregnancy for the past nine years.

Several years prior to marriage I had heard about Billings Ovulation Method of Natural Family Planning on a television program. The program described the different striations of fertile and non-fertile mucus. It seemed practical, safe, and clean, using only the body's own natural substances without chemicals or barriers to achieve or avoid pregnancy.

This information remained in the back of my mind until our Engaged Encounter where I heard of a group working in Etobicoke, Ontario. We became involved with this group. However, my husband was not encouraged to be involved in the day to day charting. This and the need to take my basal metabolic temperature were drawbacks for us.

Through Madonna House, Toronto we heard of Marguerite Bourgeoys Family Services and their use of the Creighton Ovulation model of NFP which focuses on the couple relationship. Through this method, we decided to avoid pregnancy until we were both ready to conceive. During this time there were early indicators of infertility problems.[47] These were dealt with through NFP teachings and medical involvement, initially with doctors who were support-

[47] Editors note: Charting in Natural Family Planning can be an excellent record of the reproductive health of a woman. Without the need for invasive tests, one can tell that there are signs of infertility or sub-fertility — signs such as irregular or shortened luteal phase, mucus qualities, and abnormal bleeding patterns.

ive of MBFS and familiar with Dr. Hilgers' work. Dr. Teresa M., Our NFP Instructor and Dr. Elizabeth T., Our family physician were supportive through our infertility problems, maintaining our dignity as a Catholic couple. Discussing our options was less stressful as we knew methods of testing and conceiving would be in keeping with our moral values.

Dr. Elizabeth was of great help after her initial hesitation of being involved with us. Through studying Dr. Hilgers' methodology at Pope Paul VI Institute for the Study of Human Reproduction, Dr. Elizabeth determined there were a few areas contributing to infertility and a potential for miscarriage because of hormonal deficiencies. Following a regime of hormonal therapy and vitamins, we conceived our daughter. Continuing with progesterone therapy through the first trimester and close monitoring, the pregnancy was maintained. Dr. Elizabeth worked in conjunction with my new Family Practitioner in Sudbury where we moved once the infertility question was answered.

When we first began working toward achieving pregnancy about three years prior, I believe I had conceived and miscarried early in the first trimester. The sensations in my abdomen were similar to those I felt when Natasha was conceived. Natasha is our gift of joy coming to us at Easter of '96 — New Life! Easter Joy! Natasha means a child of God. The circumstances of her conception and birth reinforce the fact that all life is gift. Our great desire to have a child could not "make" her. God wills each one of us into existence and we, married couples, are asked to be open to receiving this gift. The Creighton Ovulation Method of Natural Family Planning allows couples to be open to life as the method is natural and the decision is always the couple's — to work toward achieving pregnancy or avoiding pregnancy. Each act of intercourse involves a mind set toward family planning, putting responsibility on the couple for the gift that is theirs to receive and give as co-creators with God.

Humanae Vitae emphasizes love — love between the couple and between God and his people. The Creighton Ovulation Method of NFP emphasizes the expression of this love in SPICE (Spiritual, Physical, Intellectual, Creative; Communicative, and Emotional; Psychological) which is a holistic approach to couple relationship.

SPICE in a relationship helps it to be honest, to grow and to be intimate without focusing on genital contact. The periods of abstinence become times to enjoy each other at other levels of being, building up the excitement and anticipation of the sexual union.

Initially abstaining was difficult for us. It was a change in our lifestyle. Hindsight gives us a new perspective, showing us the growth and maturity this method enables. We are more creative in things we do together and apart. We look forward to the times we do come together in intimate union and more so now with a child. We have learned to make the most out of the moments we have alone — to talk, to discuss or work through an issue, to plan or to romance and love. I have found that SPICE adds to the intimacy of our relationship and the times we come together in the marital union, treasures where we treasure each other.

The marvelous body — A gynecologist explains how NFP works

This article is taken from a conference on bioethics in Rome given to priests by Dr. Lucia Miglionico, an obstetrician-gynecologist from Italy.

It is ironic: In an age when family planning is a leading concern for many couples all over the world, one method that has proved to be reliable, safe and natural is still greeted with skepticism.

In the years following *Humanae Vitae*, Natural Family Planning was often ignored, if not maligned, as a product of the traditionalist wishful thinking. Indeed, in Western societies so technologically advanced, to speak of Natural Family Planning can seem like nonsense. Many priests have even fallen into skepticism (here I speak from years of experience).

The natural methods of family planning or fertility identification are, by definition, methods directed at identifying the fertile and non-fertile phases of the monthly menstrual cycle, based on the recognition of particular natural signs and symptoms of fertility. Thus, they are entrusted exclusively to the woman and depend on the knowledge that she has of her body and on the responsibility she takes for her actions. Distrust of these methods derives from the fact that for a long time they have been considered synonymous with *guesstimate* methods.

Lack of information in the area of sexuality led many couples to consider fertility as an unknown and uncontrollable quality, for which it was indispensable to have access to drugs and mechanical devices. Today, in fact, there is a greater demand for information about natural methods which help couples identify their fertile phases. The responsibility for a better disclosure of these methods falls on health care workers and pastoral figures.

In suggesting a natural method to couples, we often find them fearful that they will not be able to understand the complex scientific mechanism which regulates their fertility. They soon learn, in fact, that anyone can be taught to detect the signs and symptoms of fertility — without needing a lot of medical knowledge or long periods of instruction.

First, let us look at the workings of the fertility cycle. Menstruation is the more obvious aspect of a woman's cycle. The menstrual loss, since it is visible and quantifiable, becomes the most immediate point of reference. Yet, without doubt, the central event of the cycle is ovulation.

A woman's ovaries hold thousands of ova contained in small cavities known as primary follicles. During the years of fertility, the brain (or pituitary gland) sets off a cycle by sending follicle-stimulating hormones (FSH) to the ovaries via the bloodstream.

The follicle, once stimulated, produces estrogen which in turn stimulates the pituitary gland. The pituitary gland sends back a luteinizing hormone (LH) to "pop" the follicle, causing it to release an ovum (the egg or oocyte). The LH then transforms the empty follicle into a corpus luteum which produces progesterone. The progesterone allows the development of the endometrium, the soft coating that lines the uterus and allows a fertilized ovum to rest in the womb.

The uterine cervix also plays a fundamental role: We can compare it to a caretaker who guards the entrance of an apartment building. Its walls are lined with glands that secrete a particular mucus that changes its character and functions during various phases of the cycle. When ovulation is a long way off, the mucus is dense, opaque, tightly woven, impenetrable. With the increase in the estrogen level and the approach of ovulation, the mucus changes. It becomes stringier, easily penetrable by the spermatozoa which thrive and survive in this environment. The oocyte has a life-span of a few hours, and if there is no fertilization it begins to degenerate.

When ovulation happens, the *corpus luteum* produces progesterone whose function is to keep the endometrium ready for eventual implantation of the fertilized ovum. As soon as the progesterone appears, it prompts a new change in the cervical mucus which turns dense and impenetrable as before. If there is no fertilization, within two weeks the *corpus luteum* stops its function; the endometrium, no longer supported by hormones, dissolves, and menstruation occurs.

The destiny of the oocyte is different if the couple has had relations during the fertile period. The spermatozoa deposited near the uterine cervix during conjugal relations, facilitated by the presence of the cervical mucus, go through the cervical canal into the uterus and reach the oocyte near the external third of the uterine tube. When the fusion of the two cells occurs, a new life begins.

In the history of natural methods, research has made tremendous inroads. In terms of reproductive physiology, a woman differs from a man in her recurrent phases of fertility, separated by long phases of infertility. Hence, all studies are concentrated on the recognition of the central phenomenon of the cycle: ovulation.

In the 1930's two gynecologists, Dr. Knaus of Australia and Dr. Ogino of Japan, discovered, independently of each other, that in a menstrual cycle, what varies is the period that precedes ovulation, while the post-ovulation period remains a fixed period of two weeks.

That was the discovery of the Rhythm Method. This method is based on the statistical estimate of the fertile period, taking into account the length of a woman's cycle over the course of at least a year. The great limitation of such a method was tied to the great variability of the cycles themselves and to the impossibility of applying the methods in particular to periods such as nursing and menopause, when a woman is usually infertile.

The spread of the "core temperature" method was a step forward in the 1950's. Since the 19th century it was known that near the time of menstruation a woman's core temperature falls. The successive rise in the temperature during certain days of the cycle was correlated to the activity of the *corpus luteum*, which secretes progesterone. Thus it was found that the body temperature remains low during the pre-ovulatory period. With ovulation and the formation of the *corpus luteum*, the temperature rises noticeably until the beginning of menstruation and the coinciding loss of progesterone. Successively the combination of certain signs and symptoms such as the core temperature, along with the observation of the cervical mucus and the calculation of the rhythm, led to the spread of the Symptho-thermal Method.

But it is to the Billings couple that we owe the development of a method that is both easy to learn and to apply. John Billings relates that in 1953 he and his wife were asked by a priest for help in instructing newlywed couples on natural methods to regulate their fertility. They knew about the rhythm and core temperature methods, but they also had heard talk of the cervical mucus as a "fertility indicator."

With the help of his wife Lyn and the valid scientific contribution of numerous researchers, he developed the Billings Ovulation Method, which is based exclusively on the woman's knowledge of herself and on observable changes in the cervical mucus during various phases of the cycle. With attentive observation a woman can detect the start of her fertile period, the ovulatory peak and its end.

It is a method that can help couples who want to avoid pregnancy as well as those who want to conceive. It has become one of the most popular natural methods (more than fifty million couples use it). Its spread has been facilitated by the presence of numerous training centers worldwide. Mothers, as well, have been able to pass it on to their daughters.

The Billings method permits couples to walk hand-in-hand in harmony with nature. For the woman and the man, the observation of the course of the cycle becomes a communal experience. They both live the various moments of fertility. Together they discuss the difficulties and together they find the solutions. Their free discussions about their sexuality enliven daily dialogue in a unique way. The days of abstinence or continence are not "days without love," because conjugal rapport is no longer identified only with the sexual relationship.

In this way Natural Family Planning is in sync with the life of the couple. The number of children they have will no longer be their main preoccupation. Their lives, instead, will focus on the service they can render society by their example. For the Christian couple, Natural Family Planning will become the most direct way of welcoming and bearing witness to the marvels of God's design over human love.

Surprise! How NFP brought me to the Catholic Church

Our story may not be as exciting as others, but there is a story so we will share it.

My father died when I was four, leaving my two older sisters and I to be raised by our Catholic mother. We were very fortunate that love was in our home. I enjoyed life and was cared for so well that I lived there all my single life until I was twenty-nine years old.

In my early twenties, I was seeking to know what was my purpose in life. I attended a Home Bible study, and soon started attending a non-Denominational Church. For years I attended Sunday morning and night services, midweek singles services, Friday night street witnessing, as well as the Home Bible study on Tuesday nights. I wanted to learn more about God, and also hoped to meet a strong Christian to marry while attending these meetings. But being raised in a home with all ladies it was hard to talk to men.

Once at a midweek service the preacher said, "Before we could pray for a mate we need to pray for a date." On my way home that evening I decided to take that advice and prayed for a date. I seldom, almost never, had calls from any men except my grandfather. God answered that prayer quickly — when I walked into the house my mother said I had received a call from Joe. Joe was from a Catholic charismatic prayer meeting my sister attended. I had a date! Even though I had a date, I did not think that this could be the one. He was Catholic, and I went to a non-Denominational Church. We were not equally yoked. But I was wrong — this *was* the one. Joe was the patient, and kind friend I felt comfortable being with. After dating three years we made the decision to be married.

During our engagement Joe had noticed an ad for Natural Family Planning at his Church's bulletin board. Joe was interested in the classes for moral reasons and it sounded good to me because I liked anything natural. We attended all four classes and heard things we had never heard anywhere else and they made so much sense.

After we were married, we tried to attend both our churches on sundays, but after our first child things started to change. Sunday mornings became more challenging as our child grew. The non-Denominational Church had a nursery for infants but I did not take Joanna there. We followed what we were taught in our NFP class — mother-baby togetherness and nursing on demand. As she grew, so did her noise level. The cries of infants were not a common voice in our two-hour service. Going to both services suddenly did not seem quite as appealing. It was also very hard to find anyone at the non-Denominational Church who shared our views on NFP. Contraception was just a normal acceptable practice. It was getting harder to find common grounds. So we started to only attend the Catholic Church that was a half block away from the home we had just purchased.

We began attending the Couple to Couple League's chapter meetings, always enjoying the people and views. We saw how the teaching of this group on NFP made such a positive impact on our lives. It helped to draw us together as a couple. We wanted to share this valuable information with others.

Before I met Joe, I thought I knew how I should be serving God by attending a non-Denominational Church. But God is ever surprising to bring us more fully into His Plan. We must be open to do what God wants, not what we want. I have found the Catholic Church to have something I could not find in other churches when it comes to life issues. Without these teachings, much would be lost to our future generations because they were not allowed to fulfill God's Plan in their lives.

Dare to break the tyranny? A woman describes how she did it

He is a theology professor and she is a writer, this couple has been married for sixteen years and has used NFP all the years of their marriage. They have two children and live in Florida.

I married in my mid-thirties. I first learned about NFP when I was in my mid-twenties and was teaching at a Catholic high school. I knew about *Humanae Vitae*, and fully accepted it. My students thought I was crazy and made fun of me. It was during that time that I found in a Catholic paper in Miami, *The Voice*, about the Couple to Couple League. I wrote them and got a copy of their book, which at the time was a set of mimeographed sheets.

When I eventually became engaged, John Kippley happened to have been invited by the Archdiocese for a weekend seminar and my husband-to-be and I attended it. We were both impressed by Mr. Kippley. I began charting about two years before our wedding and I was very grateful to learn about my body.

The initial motivation for using NFP was a religious one. I believed that if the Catholic Church said that contraception was wrong, contraception had to be wrong. Otherwise, how was I to believe that it was the true Church? It seemed to me that married life and family planning were crucial aspects of our lives. If the Church were wrong on that, there really was no reason to believe the Church should be right on other issues.

Eventually, an equally strong motivation kept me with NFP: as a woman I could not, still cannot, fathom why I would have to take a pill to change the natural workings of my body. I could not fathom either how I was supposed to "protect" myself from the semen of the man whom I loved, or how either one of us would ever have to change our bodies, either by medications or surgery, in order to snuff out our fertility. It seemed, and it still seems, so obvious, that the natural connection between sexual love and child bearing should be respected and not interfered with.

The Sympto-thermal Method worked well for us. There were some times when the days of abstinence seemed to be excessive, but that did not hurt our marriage. The abstinence itself was a plus, since it kept us from taking sex for granted and it made us desire it more. I think that if I had more knowledge at the time of the Billings indication for what they call the second infertile pattern, those prolonged periods of abstinence would have been greatly shortened.

Regarding unplanned pregnancy, we did not have one. Both our pregnancies were planned. However, I did have a cycle where I had every indication that I had conceived when we had not intended the pregnancy. It was a tremendously difficult three-weeks, at the end of which, with my husband's help, I had come to accept and welcome the pregnancy. Unfortunately, there was no pregnancy — only an unusually long (twenty-day) luteal phase.[48]

How do I see NFP different from contraception? They are two worlds apart. With contraception, one engages in the sexual act while at the same time going against (contra) its potential fertility. That going against fertility is like an atomic bomb that destroys the essential unity of human love and human life. In doing so, it not only interferes with the natural union of sex and new life, but it initiates a chain reaction of disunity — between husband and wife, spouses and children, men and women in general, society and the child. Sexual pleasure becomes a right first, and eventually it becomes a tyrant. It is a tyrant who does not care if it has to kill the children that are born as a result. It is a tyrant who lies, seduces, manipulates, and uses the ones who provide the abortions.

[48] Editor's note: Luteal phase is the period after ovulation until menstruation and is on the average 14 days long. A long luteal phase could mean that the woman is pregnant because her menses was not forthcoming.

With NFP, one acknowledges the intrinsic unity of human sexual love and conception of new life. The child, planned or not, is seen as a fruit of love. And when the couple realizes that at a given time, it is not prudent to conceive a new child, instead of destroying the unity, they respect it. They both have to control themselves as any mature human being is capable and expected to control himself or herself. They learn to express their love in ways that are not orgasmic. They are challenged to become intimate without copulating. If for whatever reason, a failure of the method or human fallibility, they conceive a child that was not planned, the child is seen equally as a fruit of love and they take responsibility for it.

In the US, the Supreme Court ruled that abortion is necessary because people have become accustomed to leading their intimate lives with the understanding that if contraception fails, abortion is there available to them. Abortion is legal in this country as a legal back up for failed contraception. With NFP, when all our human efforts result in an unplanned child, we rely on "back up love" to welcome that life. This love flows from the love of the couple and is supported by a loving church community. It has as its source the very love of God.

I work part time for the Diocese of Palm Beach as coordinator of NFP. At present, even though I have held this job for two and a half years, there are not that many couples interested in NFP. Because I am Hispanic, the diocese hired me with the special commission of reaching the Hispanics. It has been an uphill battle. Financially, these people are in great need of spacing their pregnancies. The responsibility for childcare falls disproportionally on the women's shoulder. The public health clinic and society in general are pressuring these women to use contraceptives or to become sterilized.

The very first woman that I instructed had an unplanned pregnancy, which I was never able to explain. The experience was traumatic for me. The child, the fifth in the family, is doing well, but... no matter how difficult is the challenge, I just do not see any other way of planning a family without having recourse to subhuman approaches (sterilization or contraception) and without harming the moral environment of human society.

We started way back in the 60's – A freeing experience for us both

Married for thirty-six years, they have been using NFP all these years. They have five children and seven grandchildren. They live in Texas. The father is a retired metallurgical engineer, and the mother was educated as a school teacher.

When we, Ann Marie and Jake, were married on August 4, 1962, we thought six children sounded like a nice number. We were not at all concerned with family planning. God blessed us soon after with our first pregnancy and the subsequent birth of our first son in June of 1963. After his birth, my obstetrician told me about the Rhythm Method and gave me something that looked like a slide rule so we could calculate my days of fertility. Breast-feeding was never mentioned as a way to space children. We used the Rhythm Method for only a short while before we decided it would be nice to have a brother or sister for our son, who was the only grandchild on both sides of the family. We were blessed with a little girl in August of 1964. The Rhythm Method helped us space all five of our children, the fifth being born on March 3, 1973. So before we had our eleventh wedding anniversary we were not far from that initial thought we had of six children being a nice number.

When I, Jake, married Ann Marie thirty-five years ago at the age of twenty-five, I was a sexually immature person in that I did not have a clear understanding of the interactions of my emotions, intellect and will. I knew I loved Ann Marie, and that I expected our marriage to be a life long commitment. But I had little understanding what it meant to live the intimacy of a husband and wife. Our Catholic culture back then was such that if a newly married couple was not expecting their first child within their first year of marriage, concerns were expressed about the fertility of that couple. Ann Marie and I wanted a large family, and I expected to earn an income as an engineer that would support a large family. Ann Marie still tells me that we used rhythm successfully to space our children, and I recall that we "had to" abstain a number of days during the monthly cycle when we were trying to avoid pregnancy. But I can only remember once when we deliberately had coitus during the fertile time with the objective of having another baby. We were trying to conceive our fourth child and on that particular occasion we had house guests. I felt rather uncomfortable even behind locked doors having coitus at that time. (It was Ann Marie's idea since she was keeping track of her fertility time!)

Ann Marie was by choice a stay-at-home mom since the birth of our first child. And as I look back on our early years of marriage, I could see that the life I led did not change all that much when I first became a father. I was not an absentee father, but much of my energy was focused on my profession, and on whether I enjoyed what I was doing at work. But now with five children in the house after less than eleven years of marriage there was no way I could not be an active parent. There was simply too much for just a mother to do.

After child number five came in 1973, I, Ann Marie, was looking for something more reliable than the Rhythm Method, even though it had worked for us. We were at a place in our lives where the five children God blessed us with required much time and energy, so we decided to begin limiting our family size. A parish priest in North Carolina gave me some information about the Billings Ovulation Method during a *Cursillo* I attended the following Spring. The information was on an audiotape accompanied by purple master mimeograph sheets. (This was before the age of Xerox!) I used the information very cautiously and we had a lot of abstinence because I did not chart regularly — I just tried to remember my mucus signs, which did not work really well with a busy family life. But no more babies came. We also acquired a copy of the *Couple to Couple League Handbook*, but I did not try to figure out their methodology; I did not take the time to do it. We were in a Bible Study group at this time and all the couples in that group was faithful to the teaching of the Church, even though some thought it might eventually change. None of us had a very good grasp of why the Church taught what it did, but we all thought the Church had a wisdom greater than us.

We were once told that it takes at least ten years of marriage before a couple feels comfortable with their mutual sexuality. We were a little slower than the average couple. (We're sure by our lived experience that this is one reason why the Catholic Church requires marriage to be a life long experience.) Around the eleventh year of our marriage our spiritual development started to change from a personal "me and God" situation to an "us and the Trinity" spirituality. It was about that time that we experienced personal conversions, thanks to the aid of the Catholic community in a small town in North Carolina.

We moved to Texas in early 1976. From our experiences in North Carolina our growth as husband and wife increased to a point where we were attracted to attending a Marriage Encounter Weekend. For me, Jake, this growth was as if my greater awareness of Ann Marie's cyclic fertility also increased my sensitivity to her as a person. For me, Ann Marie, I wanted to share more of myself with Jake. NFP had opened the door, but I had a hunger to grow closer to Jake in other ways, too.

During that time two friends shared with Ann Marie their personal struggles with being sterilized because doctors were pushing them to make that choice. They both faced serious consequences if they became pregnant. The Catholic priests they talked to told them to listen to their doctors. I, Ann Marie, was not confident enough about the Ovulation Method to encourage it in life threatening situations. But shortly thereafter, Jake and I went to a Marriage Encounter training session and I heard a very clear call to teach NFP. I shared this with Jake and he agreed it was something we could look into. On that same training weekend, two couples that we knew rather well threw away their birth control devices.

We went to training sessions for the Billings Ovulation Method and within about six months we started teaching. Our training was with a doctor and his wife who were teaching the method in the Houston area. They had developed the course materials and did all their own training. Within a year we were asked to head up the diocesan program and really struggled with the training available in this country for the Ovulation Method. However, with our Marriage Encounter background, we wanted to teach as a couple and witness to the goodness of NFP for our marriage. We investigated the training of the Couple to Couple League and asked them to come to Houston to help us. We have been using and teaching their program since January of 1980. It is a program that has couples teaching couples and it is solidly in line with the Church's teaching, and yet it is available to people of all faiths who wish to participate.

Ever since our fifth child was born in 1973, we would periodically discuss our decision to limit our family to the five we had. But one or the other of us would believe that we should not resume coitus during the fertile time. I, Jake, am sure that there was some selfishness present in my decisions at times, being scarred by original sin as I am.

But God can even bring good out of this selfishness of mine by using our experience to show that NFP can be used for more than twenty years by a fertile couple to avoid pregnancy.

The Lord has truly blessed us in our decision to use only natural methods in our marriage. Sometimes the abstinence has been difficult, but never impossible. We treasured the gift of our fertility and the five children who were born to us. NFP helped us to form the attitude that having children was a good and holy work, which is not an attitude that prevails in the US where children are often looked at as an inconvenience or a burden. We took delight in our children and watching them grow and mature and become the people hopefully God wants them to be.

NFP made us very aware of the gift of chastity and how important it is to a marriage. We strongly encouraged our children to avoid premarital sex, and think that they all accepted that message, but we never invaded their privacy to ask. God has blessed four of the children with beautiful spouses, and we are hopeful that blessing will come to our fifth child this year. We do not think the message of chastity and virginity would have been there if we were not NFP users.

We also have had openness in our own relationship that we both think is a combination of the gifts of NFP and Marriage Encounter. We can talk freely about our sexual experiences and our openness to the sexual act. It is not something we just do; we talk about it and our readiness for it.

I, Ann Marie, think NFP has given us that freedom to accept our bodies in all their phases and the frailties of life. We're not always in the same place about having sex, and we can accept that in each other. NFP has helped me to go through the menopause without fear or anxiety, trusting that the signs of fertility were there to alert me. Trusting also that if God blessed me with a child during this time, he would provide all I needed to care for that child. NFP has also led me into an ever deeper trust in Jake and in his faithful love for me. It has helped our marriage to be built on rock and not on sand.

NFP has been a very freeing experience for me as a woman. I have had such a wonderful understanding of myself. It was through the Couple to Couple League classes that we attended, and the subsequent charting that we did, that I was finally able to put all the bits and pieces of information together *with confidence*. I strongly encourage couples to attend classes together and to share in the charting experience. That was one of the great blessings of our marriage.

The menopause seems to be here for good. Still one of the lingering benefits of having used NFP is the reverence we have for the sexual act and the thanksgiving we feel each time we come together. We are thankful for the five beautiful gifts God has blessed us and now the in-law children and grandchildren that are enriching our lives.

As I, Jake, now reflect back over our thirty-six years of marriage, I can see that the practice of NFP has been a freeing experience for me. Having made the decision to limit our family to five children, knowledge of the signs of fertility on a day-to-day basis led me to a mature acceptance of the sexual abstinence. Our fertility as a couple has been an awesome gift. With NFP we had put this gift aside in reverence, and had not tried to destroy it. Developing self-control in an area of my life that has such strong emotions has encouraged me to strive for self-control in other areas, such as the control my quick temper and love for eating. This sense of achievement of controlling my genital behavior, with the grace of God, helps me not to become too discouraged because even after sixty years of living, the control of all of my emotions is still an ongoing wrestling match. I have been told that some couples reject NFP because it would take the spontaneity out of their "love making." It puzzles me why anyone would want their most intimate relationship with their spouse to be dependent on fleeting emotions. For me, NFP has helped me to get my intellect, will and emotions all lined up in one direction so that I can strive to give myself totally to Ann Marie in the act of coitus, and not just be responding to a sensual urge.

We see practicing NFP as another one of those opportunities that God gives us to grow in our trust in him. Early in our married life we accepted the Church's invitation to tithe. God has never failed us as we professed our trust in him in this area of our family finances. Putting our trust in God with respect to our family size and sexual intimacy as husband and wife has also been a blessing. In spite of a potential Rh blood factor concern, neither Ann Marie nor any of our children had adverse health problems during the pregnancies and births. We have now experienced a healthy transition into the menopause. And even after thirty-five years of marriage, we still look forward to our times of genital intimacy.

God has gently coaxed us with his gifts to let go of our lives little by little, and to put our trust in him. Our NFP experiences, including those beginning years with the Rhythm Method, have been gifts that have helped us to grow in our trust in our Triune God. Our cup has overflowed with his generosity.

It was a leap of faith for us

As a teacher of Natural Family Planning in Indiana, she has been using it in the seven years of their marriage. They have three children aged from two to six.

I am a convert to Catholicism. It was then — I learned about why the Church teaches artificial contraception is wrong and why it is not good for marriages. My husband, Pat, knew far more than I about NFP. I did not think I knew enough to have any misconception. When we were first married, we knew we wanted to start a family right away. It was after the birth of our first child that I experienced the "what if it does not work syndrome." I was breast-feeding while I found it a little difficult to understand a breast-feeding pattern. I was still able to determine my return to fertility. It gave me more confidence. I feel that NFP is a "leap of faith." We must trust in our Creator. He gave us signs of fertility to understand and to interpret our bodies. Why else would he have given us such visible signs?

NFP is so different from contraception. It is a true method of family planning. The husband gains respect for his wife in abstaining at a fertile time if a pregnancy is not desired. In teaching NFP I have had women tell me they do not feel put on the spot to have intercourse all the time, as in the case of when they are using contraceptives. There are many advantages of NFP: safe, reliable, natural, inexpensive, and easy to learn.

NFP has worked in our case. Again the most difficult time is my breast-feeding pattern after each child. I think God wants me to experience different events so that I may help my breast-feeding clients. Abstaining has only strengthened our marriage in ways we never dreamed of. It maintains a healthy respect for each other and our Creator. As my wonderful husband tells the "*Pre-Cana* couples" that we must learn to control our passions in all things, or else our passions will control us.

I see the destruction contraception is causing in our families. Thank God, the Church stood up for the teaching which cannot be changed. It is God's law. Pope Paul VI — what do we say but "thank you for the strength to stand up against the world."

Sexuality is not just a genital act

This testimony comes from a couple living in West Virginia. They were married in 1988 and have been using natural methods ever since. They have three children with ages of two, four and six. They met each other in dental school and both work as general dentists-She earned her Doctor of Dental Surgery degree in 1986 from West Virginia University School of Dentistry and he received his in 1988. She was raised a Presbyterian and became Catholic in 1988. The following is a presentation which they gave at their local Catholic Engaged Encounter which they have been involved in for the past seven years to more than 600 couples.

There is really a safe, reliable, scientifically proven, and morally acceptable method of natural birth regulation. We would like to share with you our belief that using the method is very beneficial to marriage and will enhance your love and respect for each other.

We have been married for nine years. Prior to marriage, our priest encouraged us to meet with our local Natural Family Planning instructor. We wondered why this would be necessary since we were not yet married. We found however, that as part of our marriage preparation it was very beneficial to be open to learn about our fertility and to discuss the gift of our sexuality that God gave us as a couple, and how we could more fully share and appreciate that gift during our married life. Our instructor explained to us what NFP is and is not! This was very appealing to us for numerous reasons, so we decided to use it as the method of birth regulation in our marriage. Using this method has enriched and strengthened our love for each other and has allowed us to appreciate the fertility that we share.

To be quite honest, when first using the method to avoid pregnancy, we were apprehensive. We lacked the faith that a method so simple to learn and use could be so effective. With time we felt very confident in using the method. Many people have heard mention of the so-called "Rhythm Method." NFP methods have come a long way in the past fifteen to twenty years. We are *not* talking about the old calendar Rhythm Method of the past, as many misinformed individuals may believe. It is very important for everyone to understand that *major* progress in medical science has been made in the area of using natural means to regulate births. It is equally important to understand that physicians, in general, know very little about the most recent research in Natural Birth Regulation because it is not included, in any depth, in the curriculum at most medical schools. One of the main reasons that natural methods are gaining in popularity is because of the undesirable medical side effects of artificial methods.

The Ovulation Method, which is the method we use, can be learned very inexpensively in only seven hours of instruction spread out over a three-month period. Once learned, the method is used throughout your reproductive life and costs virtually nothing. The effectiveness of the Ovulation Method is equivalent to that of oral contraceptives. Recent studies reveal the method effectiveness to *avoid* pregnancy is 99 percent; while the use effectiveness has ranged from 94 to 97 percent. These numbers have been confirmed by three independently performed studies.[49]

[49] Scientific literature to verify statistics cited: 1) HILGERS, TW, PREBIL, AM & DALY, KD, *The Effectiveness s of the Ovulation Method as a Means of Achieving and Avoiding Pregnancy.* Presented at Education Phase III Continuing Education Conference of Natural Family Planning Practitioners, July 24, 1980, Merch Fontenelle Center, Omaha, Nebraska. 2) DOUD, J, *Use-effectiveness of Creighton Model of NFP in International Review of Natural Family Planning,* 1985, 9:54. 3) HOWARD, M P, *Use-effectiveness of the Ovulation Method (Creighton Model) of Natural Family Planning,* St. Joseph Hospital, Houston, Texas, 1989.

The other side of the coin, so to speak, is that research into natural means of regulating births has greatly helped couples who have had difficulty achieving a pregnancy. The Ovulation Method is one of three NFP methods currently available. This method relies on a characteristic discharge of cervical mucus during fertility. The other methods are called the Basal Body Temperature and Sympto-thermal Methods.

Some individuals may think that there is little difference between Natural Family Planning and contraception, since both users of contraceptives and practitioners of Natural Family Planning want to regulate or "control" their fertility. Users of Natural Family Planning gain this regulation by self-mastery by obtaining internal control, understanding and respecting their bodily functions. Contraceptive users seek this control by technological mastery of their bodies.

The Ovulation Method was first researched and developed in the early 1950's by a husband and wife team from Melbourne, Australia, named Drs. John and Lyn Billings. It was brought to this country in 1972. In the mid to late 1970's, Dr. Thomas W. Hilgers, an OB-GYN physician, researched the first School of Medicine method called the "Creighton Model." Dr. Hilgers was a young resident in Obstetrics and Gynecology when Pope Paul VI's encyclical, entitled *Humanae Vitae*, was issued in 1968. He felt personally challenged by the "...To men of science" section of the encyclical. It said, in part:

> We wish now to express our encouragement to men of science, who can considerably advance the welfare of marriage and the family, along with peace of conscience, if by pooling their efforts they labor to explain more thoroughly the various conditions favoring a proper regulation of births.
>
> It is particularly desirable that... medical science succeed in providing a sufficiently secure basis for regulation of birth, founded on the observance of natural rhythms. In this way, scientists and especially Catholic scientists will contribute to demonstrate in actual fact that... a true contradiction cannot exist between the divine laws pertaining to the fostering of authentic conjugal love."

Dr. Hilgers saw the Ovulation Method as a tangible response to the request of Pope Paul VI. Since then comprehensive education and extensive research programs have been developed under his direction at Creighton University School of Medicine. When Pope Paul VI died in 1978, Dr. Hilgers and his wife, Susan, decided a living memorial would advance his vision as written in *Humanae Vitae*. Their dream became a reality in 1985 when the Pope Paul VI Institute for the Study of Human Reproduction opened its doors. Today, Dr. Hilgers is founder and Director of this facility.

The working principle behind the Ovulation Method is quite basic and logical to understand and use. We, as a couple, learn to recognize that a man, of course, is always fertile. We are then taught to identify the times during a woman's cycle when she is fertile and pregnancy is possible. We plan genital relations depending on whether or not we desire to *avoid* or *achieve* a pregnancy at various times during our married life. Successful use of the method depends upon the couple's ability to recognize daily signs and symptoms of fertility to determine the fertile and infertile day of each cycle. Subsequently, these signs and symptoms are accurately recorded daily on a chart. This whole process is quite simple to do upon learning the method, and requires only a few minutes each day for observing and recording. Using the method enhances greater marital cooperation because both husband and wife accept a shared responsibility for family planning. Also, we have found that there is much better interpersonal communication between us because the method encourages us to more deeply explore and develop other areas of our relationship aside from genital intercourse. We especially like the method because it has allowed us to truly appreciate our fertility as a precious gift from God that is to be respected, and not to be abused by an artificial device, or drugged like it is a disease.

Our fertility is not something that can just be turned on and off at the flip of a switch. We found this out while trying to conceive our first child, Natalie. It took us 10 cycles of using fertile days to achieve our first pregnancy. Then, with our second child, John Paul, the first time that we used a fertile day to try and achieve — he was there and ready to begin his life. And the same holds true for our third child, Michael J. We have been able to effectively use this method to plan our family when we have been ready. We are well aware that it is not by our own efforts that our children are with us, but they are precious gifts given to us by the divine will of the Almighty God. God has his plan for each of us in our married lives. Without even knowing it, some of us may already be sub-fertile and unable to conceive a child and may choose to adopt children. Others may see the necessity to limit the size of their family due to serious health, psychological or financial problems. What lies in the future for us is unknown and cannot be changed. But it is our task, as a married couple, to discern God's will for our lives and give him and to each other our *entire* selves, including our fertility, in the covenanted relationship we call the Sacrament of Holy Matrimony.

Natural Family Planning instruction involves an introductory session and follow-up sessions done in various ways dependent upon the NFP method and instructor. It can be used during any stage of a woman's reproductive life, be they: pre-menopausal, while breast feeding, infertility, or irregular cycles.

Using natural birth regulation is not just a "Catholic thing," as some people may believe. A majority of couples who use the method do so because of its healthful nature and lack of any harmful side effects. Please know that, at times, using the method is not always easy. When our intention so to avoid a pregnancy, there are a few days of abstinence from genital intercourse within each cycle. We have found these days to be very life-giving to our marriage because it really makes us see and appreciate each other for whom and what we are. We are not just objects for mutual pleasure and self-gratification, but as human persons who have very real spiritual, intellectual and emotional dimensions that need to be explored and affirmed and loved in addition to our physical dimension. When the time of abstinence is over there is a sort of "honeymoon effect" that makes the genital union all the more intimate and special.

Sexuality is not limited to the genital act itself. Our unique qualities and expressions reflect our sexual identity. Understanding our own masculinity and femininity and communicating that understanding to our partner is affirming for both of us. It helps us to build our self-image and support each other's self-image.

Our sexuality as a couple is in no way limited to the physical aspect only, but also has strong spiritual, intellectual, creative and emotional dimensions as well. Too often when we refer to the "sexuality" of a man and a woman who are in love, we may automatically think of the act of genital intercourse while overlooking all other gifts that each gender possesses. We need to step back for a moment and truly appreciate the feminine and masculine qualities that comprise our being, and recognize the unique qualities of sexual interactions that already are in our relationship although we may not be fully aware of their presence. These unique qualities are primarily in the non-genital areas of our human sexuality and comprise a multidimensional nature of true sexual interaction.

We just mentioned a spiritual aspect of our human sexuality. Perhaps the most significant spiritual component is prayer. Prayer is essential to the development and fortification of our spiritual needs as individuals and as a couple. Our awareness that our ultimate love is for God, and the love we have for each other evolves from this yearning for God's love provides us with an important foundation.

With each passing year of our marriage, I am gaining much better appreciation of the dignity and uniqueness of Jean as a woman by being open to all the ways that her sexuality is manifested in her personality, as well as in her physical expression. The everyday expressions of mutual affection — holding hands, compliments on our appearances, a romantic dinner and conversation, a love note hidden with my lunch, loving cooperation in caring for the children or even a tender embrace — all serve to reassure our spouse that the constancy of our love is alive and well, and *growing*! These are manifestations of our human sexuality from those he created male and female.

We both feel there is a tremendous stereotype that our society — through advertisements, TV shows, talk-shows, movies, and magazines — inflicts on all of us concerning our sexuality (that's probably the understatement of the year). We're constantly bombarded by outside influences trying to exploit our human sexuality.

We have a tremendous respect for the gift of our sexuality that God has given to us as a couple to enjoy. When we celebrate our love for each other during sexual intercourse, there is a total surrender — a gift of self to each other. Spontaneity is not always realistic due to certain interruptions over which we have no control; therefore, we prefer to plan all day for a special union.

Setting the mood in advance helps to keep the romance in our relationship. Lovemaking can be a 24-hour a day activity — let us explain that one! Since we prefer to plan ahead for our special union due to our busy schedules, we like to make a concerted effort to *make* the love throughout the day that we will share in physically at night. Small acts of affection, a love note, a surprise phone call, a special candlelight dinner, or even such mundane chores as helping with the dishes or clean up duties in the kitchen are all outward signs of our love that point to a deeper reality. The sexual act then becomes the visible expression of unselfish love, open to life and a complete giving of self. Our unity is enhanced in the sexual act as each of us focuses more on the other person than ourselves as we each seek to give more of ourselves to the other. We have found that the frequency of intercourse does not, in itself, promote the unity we seek. It is not how often we give, but how selfless we are in giving of ourselves.

People sometimes criticize the Catholic Church's teachings on moral issues on birth regulation, without ever having read the documents or understanding the wisdom and truth they proclaim. We encourage each of you to read and study the teachings of the Church concerning the regulation of births and other life issues. Please do not be misled by the results of some opinion poll taken in a newspaper or some ridiculous talk show or sitcom on television. But rather, inform yourselves with the true teachings of the Church and make your decision based on the life-giving principles of our Christian faith. We have chosen to use Natural Family Planning not simply because it is what the Church teaches, but also for the tremendous sense of peace, and unity, and fulfillment that it has brought to our marriage. We encourage each of you to learn more about this safe and effective method of birth regulation.

We would like to close with a quote by Dr. Hilgers taken from a recent publication:

> In human procreation, the human person, man and woman, are given a very special privilege. Through their bodies they become co-creators with God of an absolutely unique singular human life. But, human life is not just life, it is *eternal* life. Thus the married couple becomes a co-creator with God and the only moment in their earthly

> existence when this is possible. The couple participates in the physical and the physiological act of conception while God intervenes to create the new person's eternal soul. If we sincerely understand this principle, then we cannot help but understand the sacramentality of the genital union; and the co-creative and very sacred powers of the human person in procreation.

Using the Ovulation Method of Natural Family Planning in our marriage had, indeed, enabled us to more fully recognize and appreciate our marital sexuality and fertility as having both unitive and procreative aspects of LOVE and LIFE. As Natural Family Planning users we share the belief that creating a life depends upon three: the man, the woman, and God. The wisest of the three should have the final say.

Pioneers who started with rhythm

Married for forty years, this story comes from Nebraska. They have six children and many grandchildren.

My husband, Ed, died in 1991, following a construction accident, so I would very much like to share our NFP story with you. I am sure he would be happy to have me do this also.

We were married in April 1951, and three months later, Ed was drafted into military service. We had our first son in January 1952, the second in August 1953 and our third in August 1954. By this time we were back on the family farm in Nebraska.

Feeling the necessity of caring for three small boys, we began a rather strict abstinence routine in our marital relations. Not having any scientific guidelines to go by, we shared what we learned from each other. (Thankfully, really, for we also have two wonderful daughters that we are very grateful for.) Our sixth child, another son, was born in 1967. This time we were fully aware that we were using a time of fertility. It was during this time that we were sure our good Lord help us discover what is known today as the Ovulation Method.

Approximately twenty-five years ago, our Diocese invited an Ovulation Method instructor to help prepare some women to teach Natural Family Planning throughout the Lincoln Diocese. We learned the method from one of these women, and then began to teach it in our own area.

I feel there is a great difference between the Rhythm Method, which was based on six or so months of past cycles, and the Ovulation Method, looking ahead and using the mucus symptom for predicting ovulation. As I had mentioned, we had discovered, with God's help, the mucus cycle during our periods of abstinence, not at the time realizing it was a family planning method. By God's grace and our love and trust in each other, I'm sure it strengthened our marriage, and allowed us the use of days that we felt were infertile for marital relations.

We later learned the Sympto-thermal Method, but decided to work with the Ovulation Method. In 1979-1980, I become an NFP practitioner in the Creighton method, taught by Dr. Tom Hilgers. For quite some time I was the only practitioner in our area, so I felt pretty much like a pioneer trying to spread the good news of Natural Family Planning throughout a fifty to seventy-mile radius. We now have four more practitioners in our area, so I'm no longer actively teaching, unless someone requests my services.

My husband, Ed was very helpful and supportive of our use of NFP and also during my study and years of teaching. It was not always the easiest way, I'm sure, but our love and respect for each other continued to grow over the years. At the time of his accident and death, it was a great consolation knowing that we had lived God's plan for our life.

I think my husband, Ed, summed it up during our Marriage Encounter Weekend some twenty-five or so years ago when he said, "Our days of abstinence are sort of like a fight we conduct together against our weak wills, to better ourselves, and then to share the joy at the end." This was very true.

Some critics of NFP have a major complaint of the so-called "unwanted pregnancies" — I think in our case, I would prefer to call them "surprise pregnancies." From our own thoughts afterward of how fortunate we were to have been blessed with two wonderful daughters that we might not have had, I tried to share that with client-couples. I would like to mention, that in my teaching of Natural Family Planning, I felt I needed to help couples understand, that what might seem to them to be an "unplanned" pregnancy, could be a "planned by God child" that they needed very much. Sometimes this is the greatest reward of using NFP.

What we think, and what God knows we need, are two different things. In being open to life when using Natural Family Planning, we are allowing God to give us his special gifts even when sometimes we least expect them.

As a postscript, I might add, that one unexpected benefit from the knowledge of NFP, was the ability to face, without fear, the irregularity of the menstrual cycles that preceded the onset of the menopause. For me and us, as a couple, it seemed so easy.

Make love, not war

This testimony comes from England. The couple has been married for nineteen years and has used NFP for seventeen years. They have four children aged seven to eighteen. He is a teacher, whereas she is a full-time mother. The following is a dialogue which they presented to their diocese a few years ago.

We are teachers of Natural Family Planning and have been so for the last three years. Our decision to use NFP in our marriage came much earlier after the birth of our much-wanted first baby.

We will try to recreate the dialogue which led us to make this decision, and point out the benefits it gave to our marriage and the benefits which we hope, by becoming teachers, it can give to other couples. Finally we will give some information about the Couple to Couple League, the organization we are representing.

WIFE (W): It is twelve years since Helen arrived. Do you remember how happy we were? We had so looked forward to having a baby.

HUSBAND (H): Do you remember the problem we had afterwards? You had a Cesarean section and the doctor advised us not to get pregnant for at least a year. We had a lot of talking to do.

W: Yes. I did not want to go on the pill. I was too worried about the side effects, many of them very serious.

H: We could not even consider the coil. We knew it was abortifacient in function and both of us are against abortion.

W: I remember we seriously considered the cap or condom but to get any great reliability you have to use both simultaneously and with spermicides. It would be more like girding up for war than making love!

H: On top of all these reasons we did have moral objections to these methods, but they were only vague at the time.

W: I remember you mentioning Natural Family Planning.

H: Well it was mentioned by the couple at our pre-marriage course.

W: They did not say much about it though. I did not think it sounded as if they had any great faith in it themselves.

H: I was not too keen you hear so many jokes about it — "I have got rhythm, I have got children..." And the popular cliché of Vatican Roulette.

W: Yes, but we eventually decided to give it a go after picking up that leaflet from the back of the church in Lincoln. It sounded quite professional.

H: The course certainly was very thorough. There was a lot of work and reading. We were impressed with the introductory session, which gave us the moral, health, and religious reasons why couples decide to use NFP.

W: They did not really treat it as a birth control method, did they? They talked about spacing children not just preventing them. In fact, there was a lot about helping marginally infertile couples to conceive. The method helps women to recognize natural bodily rhythms. They understand what is happening when fertility is returning after childbirth and when fertility is fading away at pre-menopause.

H: We were surprised by the inclusion of ecological breast-feeding as a tool for natural mothering and a natural method of child spacing in its own right. I felt the importance they attached to involving husbands in the whole program was exceptionally good.

W: It gave us a very good start and the next few years brought home to us the importance in our lives of NFP.

H: It enabled us to space our four children thoughtfully, given the fact that all births were Cesareans, and we came to realize that it was the keystone in our marriage.

W: It was only slowly, in a roundabout way that it dawned upon us that all this was in accord with traditional Christian teaching and that maybe the Church was not being as stubborn or uncaring of the sexual needs of married couples as we had thought.

H: From my point of view it meant rethinking my pre-marriage criticism of the Church's teaching and realizing that with NFP, Christian marriage was in much safer hands than I thought.

W: In order to practice NFP harmoniously we found we had to communicate more fully with one another and use times of sexual abstinence creatively. People usually shudder at the thought of sexual abstinence, but with our method it is normally only required between seven and ten days in each cycle and we have found it not a hindrance but a help to our marriage. It requires commitment as well as physical, spiritual and emotional communication.

H: We are convinced that marital chastity is the right way. We began to see that it was God's will for our marriage, but it had to be our will too. We believe that a marriage is not just two people living together, but it is husband, wife and God. So we communicate with God at the spiritual level by praying together for his help and guidance.

W: Like all married couples, we need physical contact but that does not always have to lead to sexual intercourse. It does wonders for our married life to experience the same joys of our romantic days of courtship every month-being able to spend time in each other's arms without expecting sexual intercourse to follow. We talk to each other, we know each other better than ever. We are friends and our loving is very much alive and growing.

H: It is also going to be easier for us to advise our children to abstain from sex until marriage. Because we are able to practice marital chastity ourselves, our advice will be more credible to them.

W: I wish people knew what they were missing, do not you?

H: They can only find out by trying it. It is rather sad that many Christian couples are missing out while many non-believers are turning to NFP through an interest in personal ecology. They know that because NFP uses no drugs or devices, it will have no harmful side effects.

W: Also because using NFP fosters the same strengths which are necessary for marital fidelity and lifelong marriage, it could be a help in these days of escalating divorce rates.

H: Yes, did you know that one survey in the USA put the divorce rate among NFP users at 2% whereas the national average is 50%.

W: People still take some convincing though-why do you think this is?

H: The Church particularly in its medical and lay ministries was probably slow to implement a well-organized program of instruction for couples in NFP. Even in the early days when Calendar Rhythm was used it was not taught well, generally, and the failure rate then was probably unnecessarily high. Even so its failure rate is only slightly worse than the condom.

W: People are not aware that modern Natural Family Planning methods have come a long way since the days of Calendar Rhythm. No knowledgeable person teaches that method any more.

H: The Couple to Couple League (CCL) was founded in 1971. It is the largest NFP organization in North America and growing to become the largest in the world. It is a nonprofit, interfaith apostolate that trains and certifies volunteers to teach NFP in their own communities. These teachers receive ongoing support from the League's professional staff in particular, the Medical Advisory Body.

W: Couples can be very confident about the Sympto-thermal Method which we practice and teach. It is very scientific. Because it gives couples a complete awareness of all the signs of fertility and infertility in a woman's cycle-namely changes in the temperature and mucus patterns as well as physical changes to the cervix and other secondary observations-it is highly reliable when these are used in a cross-checking way.

H: It surprises people to learn that it is as reliable as the pill with no harmful side effects.

W: CCL instruction looks at the dangers to health of the popular artificial methods.

H: But more is involved in the family planning decision than just the physical aspects of a birth control choice.

W: Yes, NFP is not just another method. CCL instruction provides insights into the values frequently involved in the decision to use NFP. And only CCL instruction includes the world's oldest form of natural baby spacing-ecological breast-feeding, a way of natural mothering that according to modern research typically provides over a year of natural infertility after childbirth.

H: Anyone can be taught NFP even those women with the symptoms of pre-menopause or who are breast-feeding or who have irregular cycles (even when these are caused by the effects of discontinuing the pill) but there is no doubt that it is preferable to become acquainted with one's fertility certainly by the early days of marriage preparation.

W: It would certainly have been very beneficial for me to have been well acquainted with my own personal pattern of fertility and infertility as I embarked upon married life.

H: Husbands and fiancés are encouraged to learn the method alongside their wife or future wife and to share responsibility for analysis and interpretation of the signs as well as sharing in decisions to postpone or seek a pregnancy. This is truly a couple method.

W: The basic CCL instruction is an introductory session by a series of four meetings at monthly intervals and reading a book called *The Art of Natural Family Planning*. Classes are taught by couples such as us who have successfully completed the CCL Certification program and use the method themselves. Personal counseling is always available at each meeting and between meetings and at any future time. Finally, this is not just a method but a complete approach to married life. We now believe it to be the definitive Christian approach.

Healthy, natural and it helped my infertility

We have been married almost six years this coming August 1997. We presently live in Lindsay. Jim is in the farming industry at the Co-op Mill and is hoping to attend the associate Diploma program at Guelph University in agriculture coming this September. I am a teacher in a Catholic high school in Lindsay, Ontario. I teach grade one, but will soon be on maternity leave. We are expecting a little bundle of joy on August 14, 1997 (NFP estimated time of delivery) August 15 (Doctor's estimated time of delivery).[50]

[50] Editor's note: With the advance of modern Natural Family Planning methods, one can better pinpoint the estimated date of delivery. Traditionally, this is calculated from the last menstrual period. However, women who take accurate charting can determine the day of ovulation and hence of conception. This added knowledge is at times valuable in certain cases of difficult pregnancies where dating is crucial.

We learned about NFP through a religion course I was taking for school. A priest came to talk to us about birth control and included a brief explanation of the Marguerite Bourgeois Family Service and their phone number. I called up the number and set up our first appointment with this service.

NFP to us is natural — a more healthy means of birth control. It keeps a woman in tune with her own body and includes her husband in this process as well. Contraception to me is unnatural, I was on the pill at one time in my life and did not like being governed by medication. I am not one for pills or drugs in the first place.

In our case NFP has worked — as a means of achieving pregnancy. My "big belly" can vouch for this. This child is really a gift from God! Since we had to wait for more than two years in order to get pregnant, we do not take this process lightly! Our charts were clear indicators for my NFP instructor and NFP medical practitioner that I was lacking progesterone. I was prescribed natural progesterone. My level of mucus was low to begin with. Charting assisted us in plotting when my most fertile days were. I must admit that this was a hard time in my life. I was not always confident in NFP — near the end I was ready to give up. Two months prior to getting pregnant, I went to see my doctor who referred me to an obstetrician. He suggested flushing my tubes by a process called a hysterosalpingography. A dye was injected into my uterus and then he observed as to whether the dye moved through my fallopian tubes. This procedure allowed for close monitoring of the area. It could also flush or clean out the area. The doctor told me that many women conceived several months after having this procedure done. This is exactly what occurred. My pregnancy could be attributed to the progesterone, the hysterosalpingography or to *God's timing*. I truly believe God has a plan out of my control. NFP allows *his* control to take place, instead of my previous autopilot mentality.

The need for periodic abstinence when using NFP as a means of avoiding pregnancy is hard at times — especially since your most fertile time is a time when you are most welcome to lovemaking-the conditions are ripe! It certainly makes you look forward to the times you can have intercourse. Also, abstinence at certain time allows you and your spouse to seek other ways of being intimate (SPICE). Jim and I are always trying to improve in this area. It is ongoing and not always easy.

In the long run, I believe it will be worthwhile. With God's help we have become so much closer than we ever thought possible-and I believe further growth to endure, but all in accordance with God's timing!

A physician's struggle to do the right thing

This testimony comes from a physician working in Maryland. He is happily married with four children, Andrew age eleven, Peter age nine, Michael age six and Mark age twenty-two months.

Yes it took a great deal of effort to *confirm* my conscience — that Natural Family Planning was the only morally acceptable form of family planning. It took some personal effort before I was even exposed to *Humanae Vitae*. Somehow that had been left out of my CCD and my undergraduate teachings at a Catholic college. I did not even know what an encyclical was until I was handed a copy of *Humanae Vitae* by a priest-ethicist whom I had been referred. Thank God that the first two priests while at medical school I contacted understood what I was asking because it would be another five years before I would meet a priest who was supportive of *Humanae Vitae*.

I was without support by anyone except my wife (and of course the blessing of the Holy Spirit in strength and wisdom) during the three years of Family Practice residency that I refused to be involved in tubal ligations or contraceptives. As I sought a private practice, my decision against contraception came to the forefront. I could not find a practice opportunity that would accept me due to my views on contraception. Was my family to starve? I then had to support my wife and two children — now I have four sons. Was my medical residency for naught? I had faith that it would not be.

I sought opinion from any church leader that could be supportive. My diocese was not supportive of NFP, and the American Academy of NFP Ethics Committee was uncertain at that time (they came to support my decision afterwards). The "expert" in a neighboring diocesan office said I should invoke the principle of double effect, and provide contraception as a necessary evil for providing good family practice to a community and providing income for my family. I did not think that this was right so I contacted a priest who taught moral theology my old college and an ethicist and historian at another Catholic college. They agreed with the principle of double effect sentiments. I looked further for support of my convictions — reading, letters, interviews, etc. I knew that I must be right — that I ought not prescribe contraception, but some support would be nice.

Meanwhile, I amassed a couple of nice thick folders of information on this decision. Most of the information favored my views but every personal interview said I was wrong — until I arranged for a meeting with a history professor at St. Anselm's College. I do not even remember his name (though I'm sure I can find it) but he was important to me. He said, "You're right! If your family were to starve for the sake of your conscience, so be it. If you need to start a new career, so be it! Your conscience is correct and the double effect should not be involved." My heart felt so light after that meeting. We had walked around campus together and upon parting he said something to the effect, "It may not be an easy road but have faith — it is the *right* road." From that point on, my wife and I were able to laugh about obstacles and put-downs. They seemed so minor compared to the power of my convictions. I did find an established medical doctor who was willing to work with me knowing my stand against prescribing contraception. We have been together eight years now and have five new partners. They all think I'm a little strange but the senior partner has realized the value of my NFP care and has begun using some naprotechnology himself. And I think that the other partners are slightly envious that I am not busy with the numerous direct and indirect adverse effects (social, relational, sexually transmitted diseases, etc.) of the various contraceptives.

So I feel great! I have an opportunity to share NaProTechnology with other doctors and students. My patients for the most part, respect my position. Pro-life patients are referred to me from all over New England and I am able to help them achieve pregnancies and avoid miscarriages where others have failed — all offshoots of the teaching of the Catholic Church via the Pope Paul VI Institute in Omaha. NFP patients are wonderful people. I love to speak about this in seminaries: though I have only been invited once. I find this hard to believe but I suspect God's wisdom has it that I need to have time to devote to my young family right now. My wife has been great and very supportive of all these efforts and decisions. The two of us benefitted from the NFP community when we endured a miscarriage. They understood that life in the womb was important to us. Also, my son Mark I'm afraid, would have been miscarried if it were not for NaProTechnology — progesterone support of his pregnancy.[51] So you can begin to appreciate that the minor burdens that we have endured cannot even compare to the tremendous benefits and joys that we continue to experience.

Two African perspectives

Among the many testimonies, two came from the continent of Africa, which have a similar and yet unique perspective. Both of them were sent from the Republic of Cameroon.

H: We have been married for twelve years and have three children. I work as a nurse/midwife. Natural Family Planning was a subject in our nursing and midwifery school syllabus. I did the theory of it about ten years before our marriage. With our nursing and midwifery Catholic ethics I was already fully convinced that artificial methods of family planning were immoral and also a health hazard to most people.

W: When we were in the Vocational School the subject of NFP was introduced to us when I was engaged to my husband. I saw a lot of written material on NFP in his house, and we started learning and practicing it shortly after our marriage. He really had no misconceptions about NFP.

H: NFP as a science has helped us to understand our combined fertility which can be interpreted to enable us to live a harmonious

[51] Editor's note: There is evidence that in certain cases, spontaneous abortion (miscarriages) can be attributed to the lack of progesterone in the mother. Progesterone is the hormone that sustains the lining of the womb (endometrium). A diminished level especially in the first trimester can be the cause of miscarriage, and can be treated by supplements of natural progesterone.

life. It has helped us to trust and learn about each other and to live as equals in marriage. NFP is morally acceptable by all who believe in it. It is safe, easy to use, inexpensive, and carries no health hazards. For the effectiveness of NFP so far it has been 100% effective for us. We have no case of unplanned pregnancy.

Periodic abstinence for us both has been taken as normal. Since we respect our combined fertility cycle, this practice of restraint has become a habit. We have never regarded periodic abstinence as an obstacle for intimacy or spontaneity.

We are quite convinced that abortion is nothing but homicide, and any form of contraception that can lead to abortion is considered likewise:

Our country law forbids it.
Our religion forbids it.
Our culture forbids it.
NFP forbids it.
And God's law forbids it.

There is little for us to say on the question of overpopulation because our own district in which we live is not yet populated enough. Population explosion for us has come to mean the many jobless people and street children hanging around with no jobs and being a burden to the community because of poor moral and responsibility formation. We believe that if the world took to NFP, right consciences will be formed, people will learn to become more responsible and so bring up children responsibly.

* * * * *

We are a couple from Cameroon, Africa who teaches Natural Family Planning. We have been married for twenty-three years and are blessed with six children. We learned of NFP from a friend. We started using the mucus method first, and then, the Sympto-thermal Method to space births and to be free from risk of contraceptives. It is nature's way and therefore, it is God's way. It is opened to life — a couple can achieve a pregnancy or postpone it. It has been working very well for us. It needs a couple to become real human beings in the way of self-discipline and self-mastery. It really makes marriage become what it should be in God's plan.

"Unplanned pregnancies" are no problem to us. We have not experienced that in our own situation for the eighteen years of NFP practice. Some few couples we have taught did experience that but they accepted the pregnancies because we already taught them to be open to life in general. All the unplanned pregnancies came due to the couples not keeping to the rules of NFP and not method itself. We have mastered periodic abstinence with time. It has helped us a lot in understanding the real meaning of conjugal love. It has made us become closer to each other with a deeper reflection on our marital relationship. Thank God for NFP!

From the beginning abstinence was not easy, but with prayers it worked. The guidelines by Couple to Couple League International have also helped to fortify it. Couples should be encouraged to enter marriage with an opened mind to accept period abstinence as a gift for marriage building. To achieve this, engaged couples should take NFP as a need, as a basic requirement for marriage preparation. We are a pro-life, pro-love and pro-family. We totally denounce induced abortion, and the population explosion myth. Apart from that, all these issues are against our faith. They are also against our African tradition. We, as Africans, come from a culture that is totally pro-life.

True generosity - How we coped with a disabled child

From Georgia, this couple has been married for seven years. They have practiced NFP during all these years. They have two children. The father is a computer programmer and the mom is a teacher and dental hygienist.

We attended the same parish before marriage and knew the couple teaching NFP in our parish. We took classes before we got married. We both have strong Catholic values and wanted to do it. I have a degree in secondary health education and was curious because I had never learned about it in school.

NFP is a couple's awareness of when the opportunities to invite children to the family are and when we have opportunities to avoid pregnancy. It develops a spiritual awareness of each person's life giving role in the marriage. It promotes appreciation for the opportunity to plan a family as a couple promoting confidence in our sexual roles.

In becoming aware of the gift of life, we become more sensitive to the values of people in our society which is predominantly pro-choice. NFP enables the couples to deal with an unplanned pregnancy. They do not perceive it as a problem and are emotionally better prepared to deal with the consequences. It helps a woman to recognize changes in her body and enables her to make changes in diet or medication at the earliest signs of pregnancy.

We had 100% success. Our first pregnancy was after four months of marriage. We went out to dinner to celebrate my birthday and my wife had a glass of wine. She was in phase II, the fertile phase, according to her charting and aroused me in bed. I said, "Are you ready for children?" And she answered, "Yes." We abstained the rest of the cycle and discovered our miracle. We named our daughter Amanda Rose. She is the "beloved flower of our romantic love" and "our beautiful rose."

Periodic abstinence has not been a problem. We have home projects that we do together and we find joy in other creative opportunities. We find spontaneity in going out for dinner or getting to watch a movie together. It has given us strength to handle future burdens.

The influence of our material society and smaller families in the name of population control has planted seeds of convenience and an attitude of not being able to afford essentials. There needs to be balance in life and our contraceptive mentality has led to an over generous society of parents. Children do not work for money; they are given money and bought cars. There are material fads that pass. An example of this would be the Beenie Babies, flannel dolls filled with gravel made in China! The price was five dollars. Each comes with a card that states the doll's name and date of birth. Children want as many as they can get. They carried them to school in their school bags. Stores would sell them so fast the price went to seven dollars. Now I see plenty in stores but nobody buys them. They were quick pacifiers for parents not wanting to discipline and live with the consequences. Now they wear pets on a necklace. It is a computerized toy — you feed it, change it, put it to bed, and so on, all with the push of a button. If you fail your responsibility, the pet dies. These cost about twelve dollars and I see fewer children with them. Our society is becoming more detached from the children.

Our second daughter was born three months prematurely. I had a normal class II ultrasound at seventeen weeks. At twenty-four weeks I had an epileptic seizure and believed I had lost amniotic fluid. The emergency room physician did not believe an obstetrical exam was necessary. We were traveling at Christmas and came back to discover that the baby was not growing and there was no fluid on a class II ultrasound. We knew she was a girl and decided to name her Meredith Grace. At the time of birth, she weighed one pound and nine ounces. We believe the trials of our second daughter are fulfillment of the name we chose and a witness of faith to the people of our parish, St. Jude. Many of the parishioners visited me during her five-month stay at the hospital.

Our beautiful daughter is a profound example of our bountiful community spirit and a testimony of the intercession of our patron, St. Jude. She has been a phenomenal learning experience and continues to amaze us in her development. We continue to appreciate God's creativity in our lives.

The difference between NFP and contraception

This testimony comes from Florida of a former high school teacher who is now a full time mother. Her husband is a physician. They have been married for seven years with four children. They also teach the NFP method they have been using in the seven years of their marriage.

I learned about NFP from my sister-in-law. My parents had used the Rhythm Method and calendar temperature. I am one of seven children. We wanted to practice NFP to remain faithful to Christ. I thought contraception was for unfaithful, perhaps promiscuous or rebellious people. There was never consideration to do anything else in our marriage.

At first, I did not quite understand what the difference was between NFP and contraception. Now, I understand the world of difference between one and the other. The first person to shed light on the subject was Janet Smith through her tape — *Contraception, why not?* This was a turning point for me and gave me the impetus to choose spreading the work of NFP. In NFP, the life-giving and love-giving aspects of sex are fulfilled. We do not slam the door in God's face. We are open to the possibility of life each month. Of course, there is a sacrifice that must be made, and it is indeed a considerable sacrifice. But we have also learned that God cannot be outdone in his generosity. We have a wonderful marriage, exciting, vibrant, spiritual and communicative. When we follow God's will, he blesses us in many ways.

NFP has been effective for us. We have been married seven and a half years with no unplanned pregnancies. I have gotten to know my body better over the years and there does not seem to be any mystery. I know of other people have had unplanned pregnancies while using NFP — that's why it's only 99% effective. I have not met any of them. I have met a lot of people who say they are using NFP — but are really using the primitive Rhythm Method — and have gotten pregnant by surprise. These are people who have not studied NFP or taken a class on it. They have only learned some "day counting" from other women. It is a shame, because they still equate NFP with rhythm.

Periodic abstinence is the best thing for sexual excitement. I tell couples it is like a weekend. What makes the weekend so wonderful? It is the workweek that makes it so glorious. We work hard all week, keep long hours, try the best that we can to be successful, and the rest of the time we plan how we are going to spend our weekends. Single people can especially appreciate this because they spend hours planning the perfect weekend. The same thing happens with the infertile time. We plan and prepare for the time when we will be together again, and we have become quite creative. We do not ignore each other during the fertile time, we *date* and look forward to the time when we can be together again. Is it tough? Yes, we'd be fooling you if we said otherwise, but Jesus is with us and there is nothing that we cannot bear if we keep him in our hearts.

There is a great little book by Fr Herbert Smith addressing these topics. Of course, Janet Smith is having a significant impact on the NFP movement in the US. We have always used NFP in our marriage. Initially, I thought it was a rather heavy burden. We had four children in five years.

Then something curious happened. We decided to teach NFP. We have been doing this for a year. And you know what, the claim that the Couple-to-Couple League makes about "Building better marriages through NFP" has turned out to be true. Over and over again, we find that we are teaching couples who have been married for several years and do not want to use contraception any more because they are tired of it. They say the change from contraception to NFP has added a spark, a shared responsibility in their marriages that they did not have before. When I saw the joy that these couples experienced and the awe in discovering how perfectly programmed their bodies were, I gained a deeper of understanding of why God wants this for married couples and how magnificent is every work in his Creation.

We feel so fortunate to be involved in this apostolate and feel we are on the verge of a chastity revolution — one couple at a time. When we offered our first class, we told ourselves we would be satisfied if only two couples came. Secretly, I longed for more, but tried to not be disappointed. Sure enough, three couples came to our first class series and only two finished it. However, the next series, eleven couples registered, and the next sixteen couples registered and in the one we're presently teaching, fifteen couples. Every day, I get more phone calls about it and acquaintances in the parish timidly ask me about it. We are speaking once a month at a local parish about it, and we give talks at Engaged Encounters. We found the first people that have to be convinced are the priests and the lay leaders of our Church. With our enthusiasm and joy we can do this.

The saddest thing I have heard was a young woman who told me, "Why did not anyone ever tell us about this?" She felt betrayed that the Church would not promote this and would actually conceal this. That's when we vowed to tell everyone, because "the truth will set them free." It is often suggested that we not mention Church teaching and stick with the health benefits. The example of this woman explains why we cannot in good conscience do this.

Love that overflows – A conference of the Drs. Billings

The Drs. Billings are no strangers to those involved in Natural Family Planning. Dr. John Billings, a neurologist, is the president of WOOMB (the World Organization for the Ovulation Method Billings). His wife, Dr. Lyn Billings, is a pediatrician. They met each another while in medical school. John said that he looked up from a row of cadavers and saw this lovely girl and fell in love with her. Lyn retorted jokingly that there was really not any other competition in that place. The World Health Organization called the method the Billings eventually produced the "Billings Ovulation Method." Both Billings, in fact, have served on several ad hoc committees for the WHO. The following is an excerpt of a conference given by them to an audience of seminarians at the Pontifical Athenaeum Regina Apostolorum in Rome.

JOHN: We're dedicated to the Catholic philosophy of Natural Family Planning which is the traditional philosophy of all Christian churches. We have worked in about a hundred countries around the world — especially poor countries. We are dedicating a lot of time to working in China. That's given us quite a bit of experience of the problems of the family in the modern world.

Let me start with a story of one of our sons when he was three years old. Lyn was preparing for a party when he walked into the house from the garage with black paint all over his hands and had smeared some of it on the wall of the kitchen. "You were not a good boy, were you?" Lyn said to him. "What could we do to make you a good boy?" He replied, "Kisses make me good." He had learned that profound truth from experience.

Human beings are made to love — to be loved and to give love. This story tells us a profound truth that mischief usually arises from the feeling of being unloved. Many of the domestic problems result when one of the two couples feels unloved. The Billings Ovulation Method is not about a teaching of avoiding pregnancy, but a way to love each another more. Some people call natural methods of family planning 'natural contraception'. But it's not contraception... Because it's *not* 'against' *(contra)* the child. It's not 'obstructing' conception. Besides, Natural Family Planning also helps couples to conceive.

LYN: The method is also the world's most used method for *becoming* fertile. We have received many cases of *in vitro* fertilization which failed and the couples came to us. They conceived within a very short period of time.

JOHN: How did we begin this work in Natural Family Planning? We had a wonderful Archbishop in Melbourne, Australia named Daniel Mannix. He was an Irishman who had been the Rector of the Seminary at Maynooth in Ireland before coming to Australia in about 1915 or thereabouts to be an Auxiliary Bishop in Melbourne. He subsequently became the Archbishop and remained in office until he died when he was about ninety-nine years old. In those days it was not required of the Archbishop to propose his retirement at the age of seventy-five. Fortunately, Archbishop Mannix retained his intellectual faculties, which were very considerable, until just before he died of a brief illness. It was his custom to visit the Catholic schools in the Archdiocese and talk to the children. He believed that he could always tell which children were living in a disturbed domestic environment and he chose a young priest named Maurice Catarinich to be appointed as a marriage counselor at what was called the Catholic Family Welfare Bureau. Fr Catarinich comes from a strong medical family, his father, a sister and two brothers being doctors, and as it turned out, it was very fortunate that he had a truly scientific mind.

He took up his appointment in 1953 and soon found that many of the couples asking for help had a need to have a rest from pregnancy. In many cases these problems were of a medical character, such as a difficult labor with post-partum hemorrhage and so on. He then cast around for a doctor to help him and invited me to do so. When asked why he "chose Billings," he sometimes gives them funny answers. But the real answer was that he could see that I was happily married, fond of children, and he had heard me talking at some of the meetings of the Catholic Medical Guild which was at that time very active in Melbourne and was sure that he could trust me to follow the teaching of the Church. It was interesting also that he wanted a doctor who was not a gynecologist. This was really because many of the women were already under the care of an obstetrician-gynecologist who had looked after them during their last pregnancy and he was anxious to avoid any kind of conflict related to ethical principles between different doctors in medical practice.

At first I refused, saying that I knew very little about Natural Family Planning and was not particularly interested in the subject. Lyn and I were always anxious to have a large family and in this we were successful. (We have been married for fifty-five years with nine children, forty grand children and three great-grand children.) Later on, working in the poor countries around the world, our large family proved to be a tremendous acquisition for us. As it soon convinced the poor people to whom we were talking, and who had more than enough of family planning over several years, that we had a different story to tell. I remember in Africa being advised to talk about our children and this I did with great benefit. They realized that Lyn and I love babies and were not imposing any restriction upon them in regard to their own family. We were simply providing them with good knowledge that would enable them to have the number of children they wanted, this knowledge being particularly useful in those who had difficulty in achieving pregnancy at all.

Many of the couples in Australia had been given advice by their doctors which they were unwilling to accept, that is, advice to use contraception or to be surgically sterilized. They would tell me the story of their difficulties which were often very considerable and would then say that they would not accept the advice they had been offered because they were Catholics. I realized that I was now in the company of many saintly, courageous people absolutely determined to be faithful to the Church, and that this work was in fact a tremendous privilege and I was fortunate to be sharing it.

We realized we had to develop a method better than the methods at that time — Rhythm, and temperature (methods), etc. The Ovulation Method is a response to the serious needs of many women. We knew that God will not leave his people. We started to interview a lot of women about their ovulation cycles. We're not surgeons — we do not rush in and cut, we listen. The results were encouraging. The method reveals the marvelous nature of the woman's body.

LYN: The method we teach is really simple. Women are the best teachers of the method as they tend to be more patient and women can usually communicate better with other women. It has been shown to be 99% effective when use correctly.

JOHN: Even poor illiterate women around the world learn this method. We should not confuse illiteracy with lack of intelligence

A woman ovulates (produces eggs) on only one day during her ovulation cycle. The eggs degenerate in less than twenty-four hours. A thick mucus not only protects the womb from infection, but also blocks sperm from reaching the womb for the greater part of a woman's cycle. Hence women are infertile most of the time. Different women have all types of cycles. The cycle is under the control of the brain, through the pituitary gland. Regular breast-feeding is especially apt for delaying conception because it keeps this mucus constant — and in developing countries a child may be breast-fed for up to four years.

LYN: Couples who use the method should not have break-ups. It has been shown that while divorce rate is as high as 50% in the States, it is as low as 2% among those who use Natural Family Planning. The couples learn to see marriage and children as gifts. Many of them have come to us originally with a background of contraception and abortion. Sometimes couples come to us saying, "We do not want to have any children." We do not mind — because we know they are going to change their minds. The method is so effective that they become curious as to whether or not they're infertile. So they experiment (at conceiving). And they wind up a very happy, very loving couple — with a very happy child.

JOHN: As a man, the abstinence involved during the fertile phase when it is decided to avoid pregnancy is a way of saying, "My love for my wife and my family is much greater than the desire I have for sexual intercourse, however strong that may be." In animals, we see that their fertile periods are geared toward procreation exclusively. But in the case of man, sex implies love as well. In destroying one's fertility in contraception, one destroys the love. The avoidance of intercourse can be a means of *expressing* love — not just intercourse expresses love. When we say, "I do not want your fertility anymore," or "I will not give you my fertility anymore," we're damaging the marriage. The withdrawal of this gift tends to destroy marriages. I was shocked to notice, from the earliest days of my work to see how marital infidelity in one — or both — of the spouses often followed the introduction of contraception or sterilization.

LYN: Waiting can be positive. Husband and wife are rational and they can decide what is the best for them. Sometimes, it is a loving act to wait. When couples cooperate with nature and with each another, this generosity spills over and they end up desiring and having a child.

JOHN: Since the introduction of the pill, the methods of contraception have become more and more abortifacient in nature. The contraceptive implants and morning after pills tend to work by preventing implantation. The (IUD) spiral clearly works this way although it is almost gone. RU-486 (an abortifacient produced in France) unfortunately will be with us for some time, but as the damage it causes becomes known, it too will pass into the sordid history of these other methods. In fact, it is precisely the ineffectiveness of contraceptive methods which has led to the trend among pharmaceutical companies to make abortifacients under the name of contraceptives.

LYN: Some said that the Billings method should not be taught to unmarried couples. One missionary priest in Latin America told me, "You would eliminate 80% of our population if you demanded people be married in order to learn the method." In a town in El Salvador, prostitution was common and 80% of the town's couples were unmarried. As priests in the town began denouncing contraception from the pulpit and offering lessons on NFP, prostitution plummeted and men streamed to the priests requesting marriage. Couples' marriages and their children's baptism often took place on the same day, celebrated with *fiestas*, thereby turning the town into a center of continuous rejoicing for some time. What is more, the children of such families often went on to embrace a religious or priestly vocation.

JOHN: Another interesting outgrowth of our studies is that by timing intercourse a child's gender can even be determined with a 90% degree of success when the method is used for becoming fertile. We do not promote it (gender specification). First of all because it's not 100% effective. But also because the underlying finality may militate against welcoming every child with equal affection. Still, in China, where the Billings method is enthusiastically promoted by the government women are subject to severe penalties if they conceive a second time. This puts enormous stress on rural areas where males are wanted to work on and inherit the family farm. There are many known cases of newborn daughters drowned or exposed to die as a result. Hence natural gender selection remains a possibility under such trying conditions.

LYN: The Chinese authorities, long worried about their burgeoning population and lack of success in the measures that they have taken to control it, have turned at last to Natural Family Planning. After much study and consideration of the various methodologies available, they invited us to set up some teacher-training centers in their country. We applied for and received an Australian grant to do this work in Anhui — one of the poorest and most populous provinces. We have been surprised and happy to witness the reception of the Chinese people to the method. Surprisingly also we have talked to very many doctors who, unlike those under the influence of the pharmaceutical industries, the abortion lobby, and the artificial reproductive technologies, as are many doctors here in the West, have been very interested, anxious to learn and lacking any hostility. Already they are training their own teachers and the method is spreading.

Fifty girls attended a recent teacher-training course in Nanjing from the rural areas around the city. They are called "front fine workers" and their job is regular surveillance of the women working in the factories to detect pregnancies. These girls are very young and are unmarried. They work for a very small salary, which they are glad to get, as otherwise they would be laboring in the fields. When they came to the course, many of them riding bicycles and all dressed very nicely in their best, they did not know each other and the prospect of this course was for them a great and unfamiliar event. Very soon, they were talking to each other and were all smiles as is their nature. We found them avid for knowledge. The course was designed to cover as much as possible, introducing them to the literature which had been translated into Chinese, so that further study could be undertaken, supervised by the trained doctors at the center in Nanjing.

Toward the end of the course, we talked about the life of the gametes, and conception and the rapid growth and development of the human embryo who began life with fusion of sperm and egg. We showed them pictures first of this six-week embryo with the unmistakable characteristics of a human baby. Then we talked about nature preparing this tiny creature for survival, teaching him to suck by using his thumb to practice on, in order to develop and strengthen his cheek muscles. So that at birth he would know how to take the nipple, how to survive and how by doing this help his mother, by sucking to set in train a neuro-hormonal activity which produces milk not only as sustenance for him but also restores normality to his mother's reproductive organs.

So these girls saw the child *in utero* for the first time as a real child and one girl gulped and put down her head and cried. Many of them had to report to the authorities of any women who were pregnant so that they were forced to have abortions.

JOHN: In addition to China, couples in Islamic countries have been especially receptive to NFP. The Muslims are very enthusiastic. We work in a lot of countries where women do not receive the respect they deserve. There are countries where women are treated dreadfully... But with this method women come to demand respect and men begin to concede respect.

All this was very helpful in regard to learning so much more about the wisdom of the teaching of the Church. The fact is that there is goodness in every human person, which we must always try to reach if we are going to be helpful in bringing him or her closer to God. The goodness of every human being, not only Christians but an also people of other religions and pagans is there, but it sometimes takes time and effort and many prayers to bring it to the surface. It is love that reveals it.

In answering the question on what the pharmaceutical companies' reaction was, I can sum it up in one word: "Sabotage." At first, they ignored the method's existence, but soon the companies became infuriated, and have waged a war of misinformation about the method ever since. After all, there's no money in NFP, you know. This is followed by attempts to assimilate it. The problem is they do not teach it well and even when they do, their attitude remains hostile.

It is interesting that people with no knowledge of modern scientific NFP discuss techniques for avoiding pregnancy will often say that they have a preference for modern methods. The most modern of methods not found in nature is chemical contraception, first effected by a pill and later on by giving the medication by implants or injection. The pill was first marketed in about 1960. The Ovulation Method was first published in 1964, and so it is the most modern of all methods of avoiding pregnancy, natural or otherwise. Professor James Brown first began to work with us in 1962 and has been collaborating with us ever since. He has performed thousands and thousands of hormonal measurements by daily estimations of the ovarian hormones daily throughout the cycle, or in some cases, many cycles for many months during breast-feeding and during the menopausal and post-menopausal years. Jim Brown is a scientist and was given a Personal Chair in the University of Melbourne, with the title of a full Professor. As well as that we have Professor Erik Odeblad in Sweden, where he is Professor of Medical Biophysics in the University of Umea. We have visited his laboratories in Sweden and he has come to Australia on several occasions to work with us and with Jim Brown here. It is also of some interest that Jim is a member of the Uniting Church, an amalgamation of some Presbyterians with the Congregational and Methodist Churches. Erik Odeblad is a Lutheran. They are both active members of their Churches.

LYN: Coming back to the story told at the beginning about our son who was covered in black paint, he is now married and has a four-year-old son himself. This little boy is a holy-terror. One day, he asked John, "Do you like being you?" "Yes," answered John, "Why did you ask?" "Because I *love* being me." The aim of teaching the method for us is to help people to be themselves. It is only when they love that they will have happy marriages. And when this love overflows, they will welcome the arrival of children.

Conslusion

The testimonies and stories we have read are not only inspiring but give a real face to those who practice Natural Family Planning. Many of these couples, like you, had to struggle to come to terms with this important aspect of their sexuality. How did we arrive to the present state?

Beginning in the early 50's, there were advances in medicine that made it possible for couples to control their fertility effectively by means of the pill or the IUD. With the discovery of these new technologies, medicine promised a new era for humanity. What were these promises? They promised that the pill would improve marriages by eliminating the need to care for numerous children. They promised that there would be fewer teenage pregnancies and fewer abortions because of the high effectiveness of these contraceptives. They promised stronger families because there will be more time for the spouses and children.

Have these promises been kept? Today, we see that the number of abortions and teenage pregnancies have skyrocketed. The easy availability of contraception backfired because it allowed teenagers to experiment with sex at a much earlier age and with greater frequency, overwhelming the efficiency of the pill. Along with this comes the rampant spread of sexually transmitted diseases, not to mention the deadly AIDS virus. We also see many teenage single mothers whose future is limited by the need to care for their children. Family life has suffered a great deal within the past thirty years. The United States boasts a fifty-percent divorce rate; many of which represent second divorces.

The contraceptive technology further developed into other fields of reproductive technology. After the first "test-tube baby" was born, research has brought us to the present stage of experiments with embryos, frozen embryos, cloning of animals and possibly humans. Recently, it was reported that experiments are underway to fuse the eggs from two women to form an embryo![52] Where are we heading, I wonder?

The role of children has taken on a heavy toll within this period. While for a long time in human history, children have been considered a blessing; they are now looked upon as a curse or a burden. More than that, they are no longer considered *gifts* but become consumer products that must be tailored to the parents' needs and tastes. Parents

[52] It was reported that MIT is carrying out this research in the article, *Brave New World was only the beginning, Zenit News Agency*, January 15, 1999.

expect the right to have children in the way they want them when they want them. Thus the status of children as human persons are, but replaced to be, objects of convenience and even experimentation. Abortion and fetal experiments are the natural consequence to this mentality.

Women, too, are victims of manipulation of this contraceptive culture. While being promoted to free women from slavery of childbearing and motherhood, we see that contraceptives actually turn them easily into objects of pleasures by men who can now be freed from the responsibilities of unwanted children. "Secular feminists believed that contraception would liberate them from the chain of unwanted pregnancies. Given the astronomically high rates of abortion and divorce, it is too painfully clear that contraception has not prevented conception as it has prevented intimacy... Thus, their present dilemma: use contraception and succumb to men; do not and succumb to infants."[53] This dilemma is humorously portrayed in a letter to Dear Abby:

> I am a 23-year-old liberated woman who has been on the pill for two years. It's getting pretty expensive and I think my boyfriend should share half the cost, but I do not know him well enough to discuss money with him.[54]

When sex is divorced from procreation, the sacredness of this intimate act is cheapened. The lack of intimacy in these unions may be a strong factor in the increasing number of divorces and remarriages. Childless, without families and multiply divorced, we may see a rise of the number of women who will spend their last years in solitude. In fact, one wonders if women are less free now than ever before!

The demands of practicing NFP are real and at times require heroic virtues as seen in many of the testimonies. But *virtues* are what make a family strong and lasting. In the Encyclical *Splendor of Truth*, the Holy Father John Paul II wrote:

[53] DEMARCO, D, *The Incarnation in a Divided World,* Christendom College Press, 1988, p. 90.
[54] VAN BUREN, A, *The Best of Dear Abby,* Andrews and McMeel, 1981, p. 242, cf. *ibid,* p. 86.

> At times, in the discussions about new and complex moral problems, it can seem that Christian morality is in itself too demanding, difficult to understand and almost impossible to practice. This is untrue, since Christian morality consists, in the simplicity of the Gospel, in *following Jesus Christ*, in abandoning oneself to him, in letting oneself be transformed by his grace and renewed by his mercy, gifts which come to us in the living communion of his Church.[55]

The relation between human sexuality and faith cannot be set aside easily. The very intimate act of sexual union between two persons has transcendence beyond the mere act. The unity of the two into one flesh carries a procreative dimension which parallels the creative power of God — culminated in the coming of a new human life. To deny the fact that the sexual act has spiritual, religious, and hence ethical and moral significance is to reduce man to the level of animals.

Seen in this light, the vision of *Humanae Vitae* is indeed prophetic. It reaffirms the inseparability of love and life in the sexual act. Procreation cannot be divorced from the sexual union of man and woman. At times, love is demanding and requires responsibility and sacrifice. But as persons, we can only find fulfillment in love, for we are made to love and be loved. Only this true vision of love will bring back sanity in this confused age.

Recalling the fable at the beginning of the book, there were many who were oblivious to the imminent collapse of the palace because they were too complacent. Only the Fool, like the Church in her wisdom, foresaw the true state of affairs and sought to offer a solution — the cornerstone that may reset humanity on the right path based on the correct vision of man and of love. These stories have shown that man is, indeed, capable of love and self-donation.

Recently I spoke with a fourth-year medical student who was considering entering obstetrics-gynecology residency. He recognizes the value of NFP and does not want to give out contraceptives in his prac-

[55] *Veritatis Splendor*, 119.

tice. However, he sees that it would be very difficult, if not impossible, to go through training in the residency program to become an NFP-only gynecologist. One gynecologist told him that, "The pill is gynecology." Here is in part what I wrote to him in reply:

> When I started my medical practice in 1990, there were no other family doctors that did not prescribe the pill. My friend and I were the first to be trained as NFP medical consultants. Now, there are four doctors who have been trained in NFP working in the city. We are the pioneers. It is in a way a prophetic mission.
>
> It bothers me that in Canada, which is 50% Catholic, a medical student who tries to live coherently with his faith cannot choose a certain specialty in medicine he would have liked. On the other hand, I know of an active self-professed homosexual who went through training to become a child psychiatrist. There are many research institutes doing research on embryos, abortion pills (RU486), *in vitro* fertilization, etc. MIT is now researching to fuse the ova of two women into an embryo! And where are the Catholic or Chrstian physicians and scientists? Those who don't have the truth are pushing their agenda of same-sex marriage, abortion, euthanasia, etc. quite successfully by changing the public attitudes and law about these issues. If we really believe that truth is on our side, we too must be "activists" and not just wait for the change to occur.
>
> Our vocation as Christians is to imbue the society with true values. When we see that the culture we live in is not authentic, it falls on our shoulders to correct it. In the decision of your career, this should also be an important factor. It would be great if, fifty years from now, gynecology would be based on NFP and not on the pharmaceutics of the pill. But for that to happen, we will need many convinced NFP gynecologists willing to stick out and be different. We are on the threshold of something new and great. The question is *who* will take that first step?

This is the challenge which I am inviting to all of you who have read these testimonies. It is a calling to live out the demand of love in our own lives and to spread this message to others. On the threshold of the Third Millennium, we may well be on the eve of a revolution of love.

APPENDIX 1

Scientific Basis of Natural Family Planning

Introduction

This appendix is a brief summary of the current Natural Family Planning. It will demonstrate the scientific foundation of the different methods that were touched upon in the stories. Although much of it may be a bit technical, those with medical or biology backgrounds may find it of benefit.

History

The history of NFP is a recent one. It involves the attempt to identify the fertility of a woman in relationship with the signs and symptoms she perceives in her menstrual cycle.

It was not until 1827 that VON BAER first discovered the ovum or the human egg. However, when ovulation occurred in relation to the menstrual cycle was still unknown at that time.[1] In 1868, SQUIRE recorded basal body temperature (BBT) in relation to events of the menstrual cycle. He observed that the temperature during pregnancy was relatively high and did not oscillate, whereas, at the time of menstruation, there was a considerable fall in temperature and a variable rise shortly before.[2]

In 1904, VAN DE VELDE, a well-known Dutch researcher pointed out the relationship between the wavelike fluctuations of the BBT and ovulation. He tried at that time to bring this to the attention of the medical profession but without success.[3] Later, in 1928, he pointed out that the higher level of temperature which occurs in the later part of the menstrual cycle was due to the secretion of progesterone by the *corpus luteum*.[4]

KNAUS of Austria in 1929[5] and OGINO of Japan[6] a year later independently related the time of ovulation not to the beginning, but to the end of the menstrual cycle. Based on this knowledge, as well as the knowledge of sperm and ovum survival, they developed certain calculations which were the forerunners to calendar rhythm.

WILHELM HILLEBRAND was the first person to utilize the temperature discoveries in the practical application of Natural Family Planning in 1935. Others later involved in the development of the BBT methods were VOLLMAN (1940), FENN (1947) and DORING (1949).[7] Subsequently, the use and evaluation of the BBT method of NFP were reported in a number of retrospective studies (HOLT, 1960; GELLER, 1961; PALMER, 1963; BAILLARGEON, 1963 and VINCENT, 1967). DR. JOSEF ROETZER of Austria first began his work with the Sympto-thermal Method in 1951 and DR. EDWARD KEEFE of the USA first reported the changes of the cervix in 1962.

DR. JOHN MARSHALL published the first prospective field trial of the Basal Body Temperature as a method of regulating births in 1968.[8]

DR. JOHN BILLINGS, a neurologist, first became involved in teaching natural family planning in 1953. He devoted much of his attention to the failures of the calendar and BBT method of NFP. Over a period of years he felt that the presence of a vaginal discharge was closely associated with the occurrence of ovulation. Clinical research made by DR. JAMES BROWN, a world's expert in estrogen biochemistry, confirmed this correlation and helped establish the scientific basis of *The Ovulation Method,* which is the name of the book published in 1964.[9] DR. LYN BILLINGS, a pediatrician, became involved and established that all fertile women make these observations and teach other women about them. MRS. MERCEDES WILSON originated the use of the stamp chart.

DR. THOMAS HILGERS, an obstetrician-gynecologist from the US, developed the Creighton Model based on the Ovulation Method with standardization of the charting and of teaching. He founded the Pope Paul VI Institute which carries out research in NFP and reproductive health.

In 1971, JOHN KIPPLEY founded the Couple to Couple League together with his wife Sheila which is one of the most extensive teaching organizations of the Sympto-thermal Method of NFP in the USA. As the name suggests, this group promotes teaching by couples teaching other couples the method.

Human Reproductive Physiology

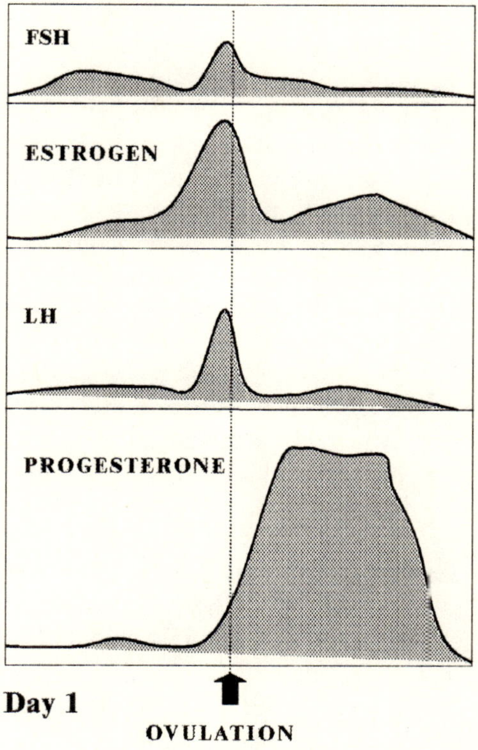

Fig. 1: HORMONES OF THE MENSTRUAL CYCLE

It is important to have a basic understanding of the hormonal changes that occur in the menstrual cycle in any discussion of NFP. The four main hormones found in Figure 1 are the Follicle Stimulating Hormone (FSH), the Luteinizing Hormone (LH), Estrogen and Progesterone. FSH and LH are hormones produced in the pituitary gland which act on the ovaries. Estrogen and Progesterone are ovarian hormones which are by-products of the cyclic function of the ovary. As the menstrual cycle commences (Day 1) or sometime afterwards, the FSH increases. This increase stimulates the ovary to develop one of the follicles which contain the ovum. As the follicle grows in size, LH stimulates it to produce estrogen (in the *theca interna*). As estrogen begins to rise, it stimulates the endocervical crypts to produce cervical mucus in increasing quantity and chanted characteristics. For some poorly understood reason, the estrogen level reaches it peak one day before ovulation. This causes the LH surge-an abrupt surge of the LH which in turn causes the follicle to contract and rupture. The ovum or egg is then release from the ovary by this process called ovulation.

After the release of the egg, it is picked up by the fimbriae and carried to the fallopian tubes which, if fertilization should occur, allows the fertilized egg to travel and implant itself in the uterine wall.

Once ovulation has taken place, the follicle which ruptured developed into a *corpus luteum* which is responsible for the production of progesterone. Because progesterone is thermogenic[10], it causes an increase in the basal body temperature, generally in the range of 0.4 °F to 1.0 °F. Both progesterone and estrogen are important in preparing the development of the endometrium which, if fertilization were to take place, allows the implantation. If there were no implantation, the drop of the hormonal levels causes the endometrium to shed in the process commonly known as menstruation. The fall of estrogen and progesterone also stimulates the pituitary via a feedback mechanism to produce FSH and this starts the cycle all over again.

There are symptoms that are associated with ovulation in a woman. Breast tenderness tends mostly to be a post-ovulatory or premenstrual symptom. Intermenstrual pain (*Mittelschmerz*) is found at times at the time of ovulation. Other symptoms are low backache, abdominal bloating, intermenstrual bleeding and vulvar swelling.

Traditionally, it has been taught that the length of the menstrual cycle is 28 days with ovulation occurring on day 14. Recent studies however showed that the cycle length is variable with an average of 30.1 days at age 20.[11] This average declines with age.[12] In fact, only 16% of cycles were found to be 28-day length in any age group. The great variability of the cycle is due to the variable length of the pre-ovulatory (follicular) phase. On the other hand, the post-ovulatory (luteal) phase is relatively constant in length for a given woman. The average length being phase is 13.7 days with a normal range of 9 -17 days.[13]

The concept of Natural Family Planning is based on the fact that ovulation typically does not occur more than once during the same menstrual cycle, unless it is within the same 24-hour period.[14] An equally important consideration is that while intercourse may hasten by a few hours the rupture of an already ripe follicle, intercourse-induced ovulation, which occurs in certain mammals, does not occur in human beings.[15]

A discussion of the characteristics of the cervical mucus is now necessary because of its important role in many NFP methods. Human cervical mucus can best be described as a hydrogel consisting mostly of water and mucins, or glycoprotein polymers. The two main types of mucus are type E and type G.[16]

When there is a preponderance of estrogen, the cells in the endocervical crypts produce a clear, stretchy, lubricative mucus-type E mucus. This mucus contains mucins which aggregate to form micelles arranged in parallel orientation allowing increased sperm penetration. The water content of type E mucus increases around the time of ovulation and makes its more elastic. The concentration of sodium and potassium salts in the mucus also increases as ovulation approaches. As a result, peri-ovulatory mucus forms a fern pattern when dried on a microscope slide.

After ovulation has occurred, progesterone as the dominant hormone abruptly halts the production of type E mucus and stimulates the crypts to produce a sticky opaque type G mucus. This mucus has decreased water content and an increased mucin content. After ovulation, the mucin is arranged as a dense network; micelles do not form and there is extensive cross-linking. Sperm penetration is nearly impossible when this type of mucus is present. Extensive hormonal assessment and correlation with the mucus change have been documented.[17] Serial ultrasound examination of the ovarian follicle also yielded similar correlation.[18]

Current scientific data suggest that once the ovum is released, it is viable for fertilization for 12 to 24 hours. If fertility were left to the random intercourse of couples to coincide with ovulation alone, pregnancy would have been quite infrequent. However, the presence of cervical mucus type E allows the sperm to survive three to five days in the cervix, hence broadening the actual time of fertility. In the absence of type E mucus, sperms die within hours in the acidic vaginal environment.[19] Also, morphologically defective sperm are filtered out by type E mucus, which prepares the remaining high-quality sperm for successful fertilization.[20]

These data points to the existence a *biological valve.*[21] As ovulation approaches, the physical qualities of the cervical mucus change. This change is geared toward the preservation and penetration of the spermatozoa. However, this condition is reversed after ovulation around four days afterwards. This biological valve phenomenon has been well shown by Moghissi.[22]

Calendar Rhythm Method

As mentioned before, the relationship between ovulation and the start of the next menstrual period was established around 1930's. This information was used to develop calendar calculations which, when based on a certain number of previous cycles, would help a couple determine when a woman could be considered infertile during future cycles.

Despite the bad press this "Rhythm" method received, many couples have been able to space the births of their children for several decades. It has not been promoted as a method of NFP for many years because women with irregular cycles, women who are breast-feeding or women with postponed ovulation cannot depend on the calendar rhythm method. Because at least 25 percent of women who present to an NFP teaching center will be classified in one of these categories, alternative strategies to predict ovulation are necessary.[23, 24]

Calendar Temperature Method

The discovery of the rise of basal body temperature (BBT) after ovulation due to the increase of progesterone has been utilized in NFP in conjunction with the calendar method. Since the rise of BBT is a post-ovulatory event, the infertile period in the post-ovulatory or luteal phase can be accurately determined. However, the pre-ovulatory phase of infertility has to rely on the calculations from the calendar rhythm which carries with it the same deficiencies. For this method to be highly effective, only the post-ovulatory phase of infertility was recommended which requires extended period of abstinence. In this method, there is also the difficulty in identifying the period of infertility after pregnancy, before the return of fertility.

Ovulation Method

Today, there exist two models of the ovulation method. The original one is the Billings Ovulation Method, the second being the Creighton Model or its new name the NaProTechnology.

Drs. John and Lyn Billings were the first to incorporate the observations of cervical mucus into methods of NFP. In 1964, the ovulation method of predicting fertility was described and in 1972, the ovulation method was introduced in the United States. In that same year, the first prospective trial of the ovulation method was published.[25] A number of published studies have been performed in many different countries since the 1970's.[26, 27, 28, 29, 30, 31]

The Ovulation Method relies solely on characteristics of the cervical mucus to accurately define the period of fertility. It does not incorporate internal examinations or temperatures. The Peak day is considered to be the last day that cervical mucus is clear, stretches easily and lubricative.[32] Several studies have demonstrated that the existence of this peak mucus, as determined by external self-examination, is closely correlated with the estimated time of ovulation determined by hormonal assay studies.[33, 34, 35] The largest of these studies[36] reported excellent correlation between the peak mucus sign and the estimated time of ovulation.

Couples monitor cervical mucus changes during the menstrual cycle using a chart. Daily entries include a description of mucus and a stamp that correlates with the description.[37] Post-ovulatory infertility begins on the fourth day after the day of the peak mucus sign. While this rule was developed empirically, the reliability of the rule has been confirmed by hormonal studies, which showed that no ovulatory events occurred more than three days after the peak mucus sign.[38, 39, 40] In the pre-ovulatory phase, a woman is considered infertile during the days before cervical mucus begins. Days of menstruation, however, are considered possibly fertile because an early mucus build-up might be obscured by the menstrual flow. Special instructions have been developed for women who have a continuous or variable presence of mucus,[41] women who have irregular bleeding and women who are breast feeding.[42, 43]

The advantage of the Ovulation Method lies in its versatility. Temperature methods described before require the presence of the *corpus luteum* which develops after the ovulation. On the other hand, the ovulation method is based primarily on the events leading up to ovulation-the absence of characteristic mucus discharge which indicates that ovulation is not yet approaching and that the natural phase of infertility is present. Hence, previously difficult cases, such as long and irregular cycles, breast-feeding, coming off the pill, anovulatory states and the pre-menopause, all can now be dealt with.

Dr. Thomas Hilgers is an obstetrician-gynecologist from the US who decided to study and review all the current NFP methods in the 1970's.[44, 45, 46, 47, 48, 49] His research resulted in what is known as the Creighton Model of the Ovulation Method today. He incorporates in this method a teaching methodology, its evaluation and standardization. It also includes the conduct of effectiveness studies, an examination of the behavioral dimensions of the method, and an extensive evaluation of its use as a system for helping women monitor their own health care. In the recent years, Dr. Hilgers also incorporates medical and surgical elements in what he coins as NaProTechnology. He defined NaProTechnology as the science which devotes its medical, surgical and allied health energies to cooperating with the natural procreative mechanisms and functions. Knowledge from the charting[50] allows for evaluation, monitoring and maintenance of gynecological health. Diseases such as PMS, endometriosis, cervical erosions, infertility, pelvic adhesions, dysmenorrhea, ovarian cysts and recurrent miscarriages can be accurately diagnosed and treated.[51]

Sympto-thermal Method

Systems collectively classified as the Sympto-thermal Methods are NFP methods which incorporate all the methods discussed above. One such model is the Serena Method used in Canada. The Sympto-thermal Method taught by the Couple to Couple League and most other teaching uses the two signs of cervical mucus and the waking temperature plus calendar calculation from the previous cycles, and these three factors used together in a cross-checking way. Users are taught about physical changes in the cervix for further corroboration, but such observations are usually not included in the rules.[52, 53, 54, 55, 56]

Some Sympto-thermal Methods encourage women to watch for periovulatory signs and symptoms such as *Mittelschmerz* pain, changes in the cervix (determined by internal examination), low backache, abdominal bloating, vulvar swelling and intermenstrual bleeding. It has been reported that these observations give additional confidence to couples using this method. Charting is used to assist couples in determining periods of fertility and infertility.

Most Sympto-thermal Methods of Natural Family Planning assume that pre-ovulatory infertility ends with the first sign of mucus. In some systems, a calendar calculation may place the pre-ovulatory period of infertility at an even earlier date than the first appearance of cervical mucus.[57]

Some terminology that are used in this method are: Phase I refers to pre-ovulation starting with the day of menstruation. Phase II refers to the fertile time. Phase III refers to post-ovulation infertility.

Lactational Amenorrhea Method

In recent years, a number of prospective studies of the Lactational Amenorrhea Method have been published. In 1988, physicians and scientists met in Bellagio, Italy, to study available data for couples using the Lactational Amenorrhea Method. The consensus of the group was that the maximum birth-spacing effect of breast feeding is achieved when a mother fully, or nearly fully, breast feeds and remains amenorrheic (not including any bleeding that occurs before the 56th postpartum day). The researchers concluded that when these two conditions are met, the effectiveness of breast-feeding in avoiding pregnancy may be as high as 98% in the first six months.[58] However, these conditions are met in only a minority of women. Since the Bellagio Conference, two studies have examined pregnancy rates among women who experienced lactational amenorrhea irrespective of the amount of breast feeding.[59, 60] In these studies, pregnancy rates of 1.7 and 2.9 percent were reported in the first six months.

Obviously, the Lactational Amenorrhea Method is only applicable to women in a specific reproductive category for a specific period of time. Therefore, to become clinically useful in NFP, it will need to be incorporated into either the Ovulation Method or the Sympto-thermal Method.[61]

Effectiveness of Natural Family Planning Methods

When referring to the effectiveness of any birth control method, one must distinguish the difference between method effectiveness and use effectiveness. Method effectiveness refers to the effectiveness of the method in avoiding pregnancy when the method is ideally applied. User effectiveness is the rate when the method is used by the couple and includes the errors of usage. "Pearl rate" refers to a method developed in the 1930's by Pearl to measure the relative effectiveness of various methods of birth control. There may be difficulties in interpreting these numbers when this is applied to Natural Family Planning because unlike contraceptives, it is used not only for avoiding pregnancies but also for achieving pregnancy.

Early studies established that both the ovulation method and the Sympto-thermal Method have excellent method-effectiveness ratings, with pregnancy rates no greater than 1.0 per 100 women-years under optimal circumstances. (Billings,[62, 63] Creighton,[64, 65] Sympto-thermal,[66, 67, 68, 69] BBT[70, 71, 72]). Slightly higher rates of unintended pregnancy (2.0 % for Sympto-thermal, 3.0 % for Ovulation or 1.0 % for Ovulation if intercourse is limited to the post-ovulatory period) have been reported by the US Public Health Service.[73, 74]

Use-effectiveness of methods of Natural Family Planning has generated much controversy. A review of studies performed over the past 15 years[75] revealed that pregnancy rates varied from 2.5 %[76] to 27.9 %[77] in couples who used the Ovulation Method and from 2.3 %[78] to 19.1 %[79] in couples who used the Sympto-thermal Method. A review of studies conducted before 1980 revealed a similar wide variation in use-effectiveness.[80] Careful examination of these studies suggests a number of reasons for these inconsistent data.

First, different systems of NFP methods were used in the studies. Therefore, not only were the actual methods different, but the way in which couples received instructions differed as well.

Second, the qualifications of instructors varied from study to study. NFP methods are easy to learn and use, as evidenced by their successful use among some illiterate populations of undeveloped countries.[81, 82] To maximize effectiveness of these methods, however, instructions must be given by an experienced, well-qualified person.[83]

Third, classification of pregnancies that occurred while using a particular method was not consistent among the studies; therefore, the actual definition of use-effectiveness was not standardized. Some studies evaluated NFP purely as a method of contraception and, therefore, all pregnancies that occurred were considered failures of the method. These studies failed to take into account that NFP can be used to achieve, as well as avoid, pregnancy. The use effectiveness of the NFP method will be determined by the intentions and actions of the couple to achieve or avoid pregnancy.

The reporting of effectiveness of NFP is not free from bias. For example, in 1985 the Federal Drug and Administration (FDA) listed Natural Family Planning or Rhythm as having an estimated (method) effectiveness of very variable, perhaps 53 to 86%.[84] Apparently, they have used the data from two poorly conducted studies done in Latin America.[85, 86] In spite of the fact that the same study showed the method effectiveness of the pill of 89.5%, a 99% effectiveness rate of the pill was cited in that report.[87] Another example is the American College of Obstetricians and Gynecologists, which in 1985 listed Natural Family Planning as having a use effectiveness of 76%.[88] This low percentage is based on two sources[89, 90] which is a blanket average obtained from unspecified "rhythm" method including the calendar, temperature, Ovulation and Sympto-thermal Methods.[91] They hardly reflect the true effectiveness of the modern Natural Family Planning methods.

Some of these difficulties can be eliminated by a rigorous standardization of the teaching and charting of an NFP model as in the case of the Creighton Model. Four large prospective studies (involving a total of 17,130 couple-months of use) have been conducted to evaluate this system.[92] Comparable results among these studies indicate that consistent data can be obtained when study variables are standardized.

Today, there is still much ignorance among the medical profession regarding the effectiveness of these natural methods despite the bulk of scientific evidence. Interest exists among women who chooses these methods for health reasons[93, 94] as well as religious and economic concerns. There is a great need for better education and dissemination of these data to the medical community and the lay public.

References

GEERLING, JH	*Natural Family Planning, American Family Physician,* 1995, 52: 1749.
HILGERS, TW	*Medical Application of Natural Family Planning,* Pope Paul VI Institute Press, Omaha, 1991.
HILGERS, TW	*The Scientific Foundations of the Ovulation Method,* Pope Paul VI Institute Press, Omaha, 1995.
KIPPLEY, J	*The Effectiveness of Natural Family Planning,* Couple to Couple League, 1998.
KLAUS, H	*Natural Family Planning: A Review,* Natural Family Planning Center of Washington, D.C., Inc., Bethesda, Maryland, 1995, 2nd ed. (First edition, *Obstetrical and Gynecological Survey,* 1982, 37: 128-150)

Note

[1] VON FRICKE, JCG *Untersuchungen uber die temperatur der Schiede und der Gebarmuttervor und Wahrend der Menstruation and uber die Temperatu der Scheide in der Schwangershaft. Ztchr. f.d. ges. Med.*, 1838, 9: 289.

[2] SQUIRE, W, *Puerperal Temperatures. Tr. Obstet, Soc. Lond,* 1868, 9: 129.

[3] VAN DE VELDE, TH, *Uber den Zusammenhang Zwischen Ovandfunction,* Wellenberuegung und Menstrualblutung, Haarlem, 1904.

[4] VAN DE VELDE, TH, *Die VoUkommene Ehe: Eine Studie uber ihre Physiologic and Technik,* 21st ed. Medizinischer Verlag, Lerpzig and Stuttgaut, 1928. The function of the *corpus luteum* will be seen later on.

[5] KNAUS, H, *Zbl. Gynak,* 1929, 53: 2193.

[6] OGINO, K, *Zbl Gynak,* 1930, 54: 624.

[7] VOLLMAN, RF, *The Menstrual Cycle,* W.B. Saunders Co., Philadelphia, 1977.

[8] MARSHALL, J, *A Field Trial of the BBT Method of Regulating Births, The Lancet,* July 6, 1968, pp. 8-10 and MARSHALL, J, *The Infertile Period: Principles and Practice,* Helicon Press, Baltimore, 1967.

[9] BILLINGS, J.J, *The Ovulation Method,* Advocate Press Pty. Ltd., 1964. (The latest 7th edition was published in 1983 by the Ovulation Method Research and Reference Centre of Australia)

[10] Thermogenic means that the chemical can elevate the basal body temperature. Recent studies have shown that it is really the presence of Pregnenolone, a close metabolite of Progesterone, and Interleukin-I formed in the *corpus luteum* which are responsible for the rise of temperature. This may explain why in some cases, there is no thermal shift even when ovulation has taken place.

[11] TRELOAR, AE, BOYNTON, RE, BEHN, BG & BROWN, BW, *Variation of the Human Menstrual Cycle through Reproductive Life, Int J Fertil,* 1970, 12: 77-126.

[12] CHIAZZE, L JR, BRAYER FT, MACISCO, JJ JR, PARKER, MP & DUFFY, BJ, *The Length and Variability of the Human Menstrual Cycle,* JAMA 1968, 203:377-80.

[13] HILGERS, TW, ABRAHAM, GE & CAVANAGH, D, *Natural Family Planning I — The Peak Symptom and Estimated Time of Ovulation, Obstet Gynecol,* 1978, 52: 575-82.

[14] HILGERS, TW, *Coitus Induced Ovulation and Double Ovulation, in Reproductive Anatomy and Physiology for the Natural Family Planning Practitioner,* Omaha, Nebraska, Creighton University Natural Family Planning Education and Research Center, 1981: 45-6

[15] *Ibid.*

[16] For the sake of simplicity, this model of types E and G mucus is followed here. More recent studies have shown that type E mucus is better characterized by S-Mucus and L-Mucus. Other than these two and the Type G mucus (G-mucus), P-Mucus and F-Mucus are also described. See ODEBLAD, E, *The Discovery of Different Types of Cervical Mucus and the Billings Ovulation Method, Bulletin of the NFP Council of Victoria,* Sept., 1994, 21: 3-24.

[17] See BORWN, JB, HARRISSON, P, SMITH, MA, et al, *Correlation Between the Mucus Symptoms and the Hormonal Markers of Fertility Throughout Reproductive Life,* Ovulation Method Research Centre of Australia, Melbourne, Victoria, Australia, 1981. BILLINGS, EL, BILLINGS, JJ, BROWN, JB, et al, *Symptoms and Hormonal Changes Accompanying Ovulation, The Lancet,* Feb. 5, 1972, pp. 282-4. CORTESI, S, RIGONI, G, ZEN, F, et al, *Correlation of Plasma Gonadatropins and Ovarian Steroid Pattern with Symptomatic Changes in Cervical Mucus During the Menstrual Cycle in Normal Cycling Women, Contraception,* 1981, 23: 635-641.

[18] See LEADER, A, WISEMAN, D & TAYLOR, PJ, *The Prediction of Ovulation: A Comparison of the Basal Body Temperature Graph, Cervical Mucus Score and Real-time Pelvic Ultrasonography, Fertility and Sterility,* 1985, 43: 385-8. NULSEN, J , WHEELER, C, AUSMANAS, M, et al, *Cervical Mucus Changes in Relation to Urinary Luteinizing Hormone, Fertility and Sterility,* 1987, 48: 783-786.DAILY, DC, REUTER, K, COHEN S, et al, *Follicle Size by Ultrasound versus Cervical Mucus Quality: Normal and Abnormal Patterns in Spontaneous Cycles, Fertility and Sterility,* 1989, 51: 589-603.

[19] FERIN, JT & JOHANSSON, EDB, *Ovulation Detection in Human Reproduction: Conception and Contraception,* (HAFEZ, ESE & EVANS, TN, eds.), Harper and Row, Hagerstown, Maryland, 1973.

[20] KATZ, DE, *Human Cervical Mucus: Research Update, Am J Obstet Gynecol,* 1991, 165(6 Pt 2): 1984-6.

[21] In 1972, a WHO colloquium on the topic of *Cervical Mucus and Human Reproduction* likened the uterine cervix to that of a "biological valve" which, "at certain periods during the reproductive cycle allows the entry of sperm into the uterus, and at other times bars their admission." From *Cervical Mucus: Present State of Knowledge,* World Health Organization — Colloquium, Published Proceedings, Geneva, Switzerland, 1972.

[22] MOGHISSI, KS, SYNER, FN & EVANS, TN, A *Composite Picture of the Menstrual Cycle, Am J Obstet Gynecol.,* 114:405, 1972.

[23] HILGERS, TW, *Methods of Natural Family Planning in Reproductive Anatomy and Physiology for the Natural Family Planning Practitioner,* Omaha, Nebraska, Creighton University Natural Family Planning Education and Research Center, 1981:49.

24 DOUD, J, *Use-effectiveness of the Creighton Model of NFP, Int Rev Nat Fam Plann,* 1985, 9:54-72.

25 WEISSMANN, MC, FOLIAKI, L, BILLINGS, EL & BILLINGS, JJ, *A Trial of the Ovulation Method of Family Planning in Tonga, Lancet* 1972, 2(781): 813-6.

26 DOUD, J, Use-effectiveness of the Creighton Model of NFP, Int Rev Nat Fam Plann, 1985, 9:54-72.

27 WADE, ME, MCCARTHY, P, BRAUNSTEIN, GD, ABERNATHY, JR, SUCHINDRAN, CM, HARRIS, GS, et al, *A Randomized Prospective Study of the Use-effectiveness of Two methods of Natural Family Planning, Am J Obstet Gynecol,* 1981, 141: 368-76.

28 MEDINA JE, CIFUENTES A, ABERNATHY JR, SPIELER JM & WADE ME, *Comparative Evaluation of Two Methods of Natural Family Planning in Columbia, Am J Obstet Gynecol* 1980, 138: 1142-7.

29 WORLD HEALTH ORGANIZATION, *A Prospective Multicentre Trial of the Ovulation Method of Natural Family Planning II — The Effectiveness Phase, Fertil Steril,* 1981, 36:591-8.

30 THAPA, S, WONG, MV, LAMPE, PG, PIETOJO, H & SOEJOENOES, A, *Efficacy of Three Variations of Periodic Abstinence for Family Planning in Indonesia, Stud Fam Plann,* 1990, 21: 327-34.

31 FEHRING, RJ, LAWRENCE, D & PHILPOT, C, *Use effectiveness of the Creighton Model Ovulation Method of Natural Family Planning, J Obstet Gynecol Neonatal Nurs,* 1994, 23: 303-9.

32 In the Creighton Model, the last day of the mucus discharge that is clear, stretchy or lubricative is identified as the Peak Symptom or Peak Day. In the Billings Method, the peak mucus sign is defined as the last day of sensation of lubricative mucus.

33 HILGERS, TW, ABRAHAM, GE & CAVANAGH, D, *Natural Family Planning I — The Peak Symptom and Estimated Time of Ovulation, Obstet Gynecol,* 1978, 52: 575-82.

34 BILLINGS, EL, BROWN, JB, BILLINGS, JJ & BURGER, HG, *Symptoms and Hormonal Changes Accompanying Ovulation, Lancet,* 1972,1(745): 282-4.

35 CASEY, JH, *The Correlation between Midcycle Hormonal Profiles, Cervical Mucus and Ovulation in Normal Women* in SANTAMARIA JN, BILLINGS JJ, eds, *Human Love and Human Life,* Melbourne, Australia: Polding, p 68-71, 1979.

36 HILGERS, TW, et al, *Natural Family Planning I — The Peak Symptom and Estimated Time of Ovulation.*

37 In the Creighton Model Fertility Care System, charting is termed NaProTracking. Knowledge for NaProTrackng allows for evaulating, monitoring and maintenance of gynecological health.

38 See note 36.

39 BILLINGS, EL, BROWN, JB, BILLINGS, JJ & BURGER, HG, *Symptoms and Hormonal Changes Accompanying Ovulation, Lancet,* 1972,1(745): 282-4.

40 CASEY, JH, *The Correlation between Midcycle Hormonal Profiles, Cervical Mucus and Ovulation in Normal Women* in SANTAMARIA JN, BILLINGS JJ, eds, *Human Love and Human Life,* Melbourne, Australia: Polding, p 68-71, 1979.

41 Continuous mucus is due to vaginal discharges, they are not truly mucus.

42 BILLINGS, EL, BILLINGS, JJ & CATARINICH, M, *Billings Atlas of the Ovulation Method: the Mucus Patterns of Fertility and Infertility,* Melbourne, Ovulation Method Research and Reference Centre of Australia, 19895.

43 HILGERS, TW, DALY, KD, HILGERS, SK & PREBIL, AM, *The Ovulation Method of Natural Family Planning: a Standardized, Case Management Approach to Teaching,*

Book one: Basic Teaching Skills, Omaha, Nebraska, Creighton University Natural Family Planning Education and Research Center, 1982.

[44] HILGERS, TW, ABRAHAM, GE & CAVANAGH, D, *Natural Family Planning I — The Peak Symptom and Estimated Time of Ovulation, Obstet Gynecol,* 1978, 52: 575-82.

[45] HILGERS, TW & BAILEY, AJ, *Natural Family Planning II — The Basal Body Temperature and Estimated Time of Ovulation, Obstet Gynec,* 1980, 52: 333.

[46] HILGERS, TW & PREBIL, AM, *The Ovulation Method-Vulvar Observations as an Index of Fertility/Infertility, Obstet Gynec,* 1979, 53:,12-22.

[47] HILGERS, TW, DALY, KD, PREBIL, AM & HILGERS, SK, *Natural Family Planning III — Intermenstrual Symptoms and Estimated Time of Ovulation, Obstet Gynec,* 1981, 58: 152-5.

[48] HILGERS, TW, BAILY, AJ & PREBIL, AM, *Natural Family Planning IV — The Identification of Postovulatory Infertility, Obstet Gynec,* 1981, 58:345.

[49] HILGERS, TW & STANFORD, JB, *Creighton Model NaProEducation Technology for Avoiding Pregnancy: Use Effectiveness, J Reprod Med,* 1998, 43: 495-502.

[50] New terminology in the Creighton Model Fertility Care System for charting is "NaProTracking."

[51] HILGERS, TW, *Medical Application of Natural Family Planning — A Contemporary Approach to Women's Health,* Pope Paul VI Institute, 1991.

[52] WADE, ME, MCCARTHY, P, BRAUNSTEIN, GD, ABERNATHY, JR, SUCHINDRAN, CM, HARRIS, GS, et al, *A Randomized Prospective Study of the Use-effectiveness of Two methods of Natural Family Planning, Am J Obstet Gynecol,* 1981, 141: 368-76.

[53] MEDINA JE, CIFUENTES A, ABERNATHY JR, SPIELER JM & WADE ME, *Comparative Evaluation of Two Methods of Natural Family Planning in Columbia, Am J Obstet Gynecol* 1980, 138: 1142-7.

[54] RICE, FJ, LANCTOT, CA & GARCIA-DEVESA, C, *Effectiveness of the Sympto-thermal Method of Natural Family Planning: an International Study, Int J Fertil,* 1988, 3326: 222-30.

[55] BARBATO, M & BERTOLOTTI, G, *Natural Methods for Fertility Control: A Prospective Study, Int J Fertil,* 1988, 33 (Suppl):48-51.

[56] FRANK-HERRMANN, P, FREUNDL G, BAUR, S, BREMME, M, DORING, GK, GODEHARDT, EA, et al, *Effectiveness and Acceptability of the Sympto-thermal Method of Natural Family Planning in Germany, Am J Obstet Gynecol,* 1991,165: 2052-4.

[57] ROETZER J, *Supplemented Basal Body Temperature and Regulation of Conception, Arch Gynakol,* 1968, 206: 195-214.

[58] KENNEDY, KI, RIVERA, R & MCNEILLY, AS, *Consensus Statement on the Use of Breastfeeding as a Family Planning Method, Contraception,* 1989, 39: 477-96.

[59] SHORT, RV, LEWIS, PR, RENFREE, MB & SHAW, G, *Contraceptive Effects of Extended Lactational Amenorrhoea: Beyond the Bellagio Consensus, Lancet,* 1991, 337: 715-7.

[60] KENNEDY, KI & VISNESS, CM, *Contraceptive Efficacy of Lactational Amenorrhoea, Lancet,* 1992, 339: 227-30.

[61] GROSS, BA, *Is the Lactational Amenorrhea Method a Part of Natural Family Planning? Biology and policy, Am J Obstet Gynecol,* 1991, 165: 2014-9.

[62] ZHANG, DW & XU, JX, *The Effectiveness of the Ovulation Method Used by 688 Couples in Shanghai,* Shanghai Municipal Family Planning Commission. Presented at the Eleventh Annual Meeting of the American Academy of Natural Family Planning, July 1991, Charleston, West Virginia.

63 WEISSMANN, MC, FOLIAKI, L, BILLINGS, EL & BILLINGS, JJ, *A Trial of the Ovulation Method of Family Planning in Tonga, Lancet* 1972, 2(781): 813-6.

64 DOUD, J, *Use-effectiveness of the Creighton Model of NFP, Int Rev Nat Fam Plann,* 1985, 9:54-72.

65 FEHRING, RJ, LAWRENCE, D & PHILPOT, C, *Use effectiveness of the Creighton Model Ovulation Method of Natural Family Planning, J Obstet Gynecol Neonatal Nurs,* 1994, 23: 303-9.

66 WADE, ME, MCCARTHY, P, BRAUNSTEIN, GD, ABERNATHY, JR, SUCHINDRAN, CM, HARRIS, GS, et al, *A Randomized Prospective Study of the Use-effectiveness of Two methods of Natural Family Planning, Am J Obstet Gynecol,* 1981, 141: 368-76.

67 RICE, FJ, LANCTOT, CA & GARCIA-DEVESA, C, *Effectiveness of the Sympto-thermal Method of Natural Family Planning: an International Study, Int J Fertil,* 1988, 26: 3: 222-30.

68 RICE, FJ & LANCTOT, CA, *Results of a Recent Study of the Sympto-Thermal Method of Natural Family Planning, Linacre Quarterly,* 1978, 45: 388-391.

69 ROETZER, J, *The Sympto-Thermal Method: Ten Years of Change, Linacre Quarterly,* 1978, 45:4-370.

70 ROETZER, J, *Supplemented Basal Body Temperature and Regulation of Conception, Arch Gynakol,* 1968, 206: 195-214.

71 DORING, GK, *The Reliability of Temperature Records as a Method of Contraception,* (Uber die Zuverlassigkeit der Temperaturmethode Zur Empfangnisverhutung) Deutsche medizinische Wochenschrift, 92:23, pp. 1055-1061, 1967, abstracted in *1968 Yearbook of Obstetrics and Gynecology,* p 354.

72 VINCENT, B. et al., *Methode Thermique a et Contraception: Approaches medicale et psychosociologique,* Masson, Paris, 1967, 52-73.

73 U.S. PUBLIC HEALTH SERVICE, *Counseling to Prevent Unintended Pregnancy, Am Fam Physician,* 1994, 50: 971-4.

74 HATCHER, RA, ed., *Contraceptive Technology,* New York: Irvington, 199416.

75 KAMBIC, RT, *Natural Family Planning Use-effectiveness and Continuation, Am J Obstet Gynecol,* 1991, 165 (6 Pt 2): 2046-8.

76 HILGERS, TW & STANFORD, JB, *Creighton Model NaProEducation Technology for Avoiding Pregnancy: Use Effectiveness, J Reprod Med,* 1998, 43: 495-502.

77 WORLD HEALTH ORGANIZATION, *A Prospective Multicentre Trial of the Ovulation Method of Natural Family Planning II - The Effectiveness Phase, Fertil Steril,* 1981, 36:591-8.

78 FRANK-HERRMANN, P, FREUNDL G, BAUR, S, BREMME, M, DORING, GK, GODEHARDT, EA, et al, *Effectiveness and Acceptability of the Sympto-thermal Method of Natural Family Planning in Germany, Am J Obstet Gynecol,* 1991,165: 2052-4.

79 WADE, ME, MCCARTHY, P, BRAUNSTEIN, GD, ABERNATHY, JR, SUCHINDRAN, CM, HARRIS, GS, et al, *A Randomized Prospective Study of the Use-effectiveness of Two methods of Natural Family Planning, Am J Obstet Gynecol,* 1981, 141: 368-76.

80 HILGERS, TW, *A Critical Evaluation of Effectiveness Studies in Natural Family Planning in Proceedings of An International Symposium on Natural Family Planning sponsored by the World Health Organization,* Dublin, Ireland, 1979: 94-109.

81 KAMBIC, RT, *Natural Family Planning Use-effectiveness and Continuation, Am J Obstet Gynecol,* 1991, 165 (6 Pt 2): 2046-8.

82 RYDER, RE, *Natural Family Planning: Effective Birth Control supported by the Catholic Church,* BMJ, 1993, 307: 723-6.

[83] *Ibid.*

[84] WILLIS, J, *Comparing Contraceptives, FDA Consumer,* 1985, 19: 28-35.

[85] JARAMILLO-GOMEZ, M & LONDONO, JB, Rhythm: *A Hazardous Contraceptive Method, Demography,* 1968, 5: 433-438.

[86] MEDINA, JE, CIFUENTES, A, ABERNATHY, JR, SPIELER, JM & WADE, ME, *Comparative Evaluation of Two Methods of Natural Family Planning in Columbia, Am J Obstet Gynecol* 1980, 138: 1142-7.

[87] As the authors reported, "The results of this study indicate that these two methods of NFP cannot be considered as simple methods of family planning but as a new way of life which requires changes in sexual behavior cannot be achieved in a short period of time... The degree of motivation toward following periodic abstinence is related to cultural factors that make abstinence difficult to practice in Colombia." Precisely, this was also demonstrated in the five-nation study (see note 79 on WADE, et al.) in which the results from Colombia were so markedly different from the North American, European, and Asian figures that they were treated separately. It is unfair to write for a North American audience and quote only the Colombian studies and ignore the North American and European studies which are far more relevant.

[88] THE AMERICAN COLLEGE OF OBSTETRICIANS AND GYNECOLOGISTS, *Benefits, Risks & Effectiveness of Contraception,* 1985.

[89] SCHIRM, AL, et al, *Contraceptive Failure in the United States: The Impact of Social, Economic and Demographic Factors, Family Planning Perspectives,* 1982, 14: 68-75.

[90] HATCHER, RA, ed., *Contraceptive Technology,* New York: Irvington, 1994[16].

[91] In the first source, a publication of Planned Parenthood, the authors attempted a generalized approach to all methods of birth control employing information from two retrospective surveys in 1973 and 1976 where their failure rate for "rhythm" was 23.7%. "Rhythm" was unspecified in these two surveys. The second source was Robert A. Hatcher's *Contraceptive Technology* (see previous note) where effectiveness rates for ten different systems of NFP from calendar only to temperature-only, mucus-only, and Sympto-thermal were listed. The effectiveness rates ranged from 70% (calendar-only) to 99.7% (Phase III only, temperature-only). Thus the ACOG settled for this pregnancy rate of 24% from the first source, which is also quoted by Hatcher. This pregnancy rate is a completely unspecified and catchall "rhythm" and does not seriously represent the effectiveness of the various modern NFP methods.

[92] HILGERS, TW & STANFORD, JB, *Creighton Model NaProEducation Technology for Avoiding Pregnancy: Use Effectiveness, J Reprod Med,* 1998, 43: 495-502

[93] FREUNDL, G, FRANK, P, BAUER, S & DORING, G, *Demographic Study on the Family Planning Behaviour of the German Population: the Importance of Natural Methods, Int J Fertil,* 1988, 33 (Suppl): 54-8.

[94] STANFORD, JB, LEMAIRE, JC & FOX, A, *Interest in Natural Family Planning among Female Family Practice Patients, Fam Pract Res J,* 1994, 14: 237-49.

APPENDIX 2

Natural Family Planning Centers and Organizations

This appendix serves to provide organizations primarily found in North America which support or teach the various NFP methods. For those interested in centers from other countries, they can contact the head office of these organizations.

SYMPTO-THERMAL METHODS

Couple to Couple League International, Inc.

The Couple to Couple League
John F Kippley, President
4290 Delhi Pike
PO Box 111184
Cincinnati, OH 45211
Tel: (513) 471-2000
Fax: (513) 557-2449
Email: **ccli@ccli.org**
Internet: **www.ccli.org**

Serena Method

Bob and Armanda Bremner
340 Black Thorn Street
Oshawa, Ontario
L1K 1K9
Canada
Tel: (905) 725-2719
Internet: **www.serena.ca**

OVULATION METHOD

Billings Ovulation Method

HEAD OFFICE in AUSTRALIA
Drs John and Evelyn Billings
Melbourne Billings Family Life Centre
39 Wellington Street
Kew 3101,
Victoria, Australia
Phone: 613-9853-4121 / Fax: 613-9482-4208
E-mail: **billings@ozemail.com.au**
Internet: **www.woomb.org**

NORTH AMERICA
Billings Ovulation Method Association (BOMA)-USA
316 North 7th Avenue
Saint Cloud, MN 56303-3631
Phone: 1-888-637-6371, 320-252-2100 / Fax: 320-252-2877
E-mail: **sek@gw.stcdio.org**
Internet: **www.bona-usa.org**

Family of the Americas Foundation
Mrs Mercedes Wilson, Executive Director
PO Box 1170
Dunkirk, MD 20754
Tel: 301-627-3346
Fax: 627-0847
E-mail: **family@upbeat.com**
Internet: **www.familyplanning.net**

Creighton Model Fertility Care System - HEAD OFFICE
Pope Paul VI Institute for the Study of Human Reproduction
Dr Thomas Hilgers, Director
6901 Mercy Road, Omaha, NE 68106-2604 - USA
Tel: (402) 390-6600
Fax: (402) 390-9851
E-mail: **popepaul@mitec.net**
Internet: **www.popepaulvi.com**

OTHER NFP SUPPORTING ORGANIZATIONS

AMERICAN LIFE LEAGUE (ALL)
Julie Brown, President - Box 1350 - Stafford, VA 22555
Tel: 540-659-4171 / Fax: 659-2586
www.all.org

CATHOLIC MEDICAL ASSOCIATION
850 Elm Grove Rd - Elm Grove, WI 53122
Tel: 414-784-3435 / Fax: 782-8788
E-mail: **nfcpg@aol.com**

HUMAN LIFE INTERNATIONAL
4 Family Life - Front Royal, VA 22630
Tel: 540-635-7884 / Fax: 622-2838
E-mail: **hli@hli.org**
www.hli.org

PRIESTS FOR LIFE
PO Box 307 - Port Chester, NY 10573
Tel: 914-937-8243 / Fax: 937-9207
www.priestsforlife.org

PHARMACISTS FOR LIFE INTERNATIONAL
P.O: Box 1281 - Powell, OH 43065-1281
Tel: 1-800-227-8359, 740-881-5520 / Fax: 740-667-2447
E-mail: **pfli@pfli.org**
www.pfli.org

NATURAL FAMILY PLANNING OUTREACH
Fr Daniel McCaffrey, STD - Archdiocese of Oklahoma City -
3366 NW Expressway, Bldg D #630 - Oklahoma City, OK 76112
Tel: 405-942-4084, 1-888-NFP-6383 / Fax: 405-942-4022
E-mail: **nfpoutreach@worldnet.att.net**
www.nfpoutreach.org

ONE MORE SOUL
Steve Koob, Director - 616 Five Oaks Ave - Dayton, OH 45406
Tel: 1-800-307-7685, 937-279-5433 / Fax: 279-2370
E-mail: **OMSoul@juno.com**
www.OMSoul.com

NORTHWEST FAMILY SERVICES, INC.
4805 NE Glisan Street - Portland, OR 97213
Tel: 503-215-6377 / Fax: 215-6940
www.nwfs.org

NATIONAL CONFERENCE OF CATHOLIC BISHOPS
Diocesan Development Program for NFP - 3211 Fourth St, NE - Washington, DC 20017
Tel: 202-541-3240, 202-541-3054
www.nccbuscc.org/prolife/issues/nfp

THE GIFT FOUNDATION
Steve Habishon, Director - PO Box 95, Carpentersville - IL 60110
Tel: 847-844-1167 / Fax: 847-844-1195
www.giftfoundation.org

APPENDIX 3

References and Books of Interest

This reading list is by no means exhaustive. It is meant for those interested in further reading on this subject. Most of these books can be ordered from a local Catholic bookstore or from the NFP organizations listed in Appendix 2.

CHURCH DOCUMENTS

Humanae Vitae (On the Transmission of Human Life)
Pope Paul VI
The 1968 encyclical dealing with the transmission of human life based on authentic human sexuality.

Evangelium Vitae (The Gospel of Life)
Pope John Paul II
The 1995 encyclical which explains the Church's teaching of the value of human life from conception to natural death.

Familiaris Consortio (The Role of the Christian Family in the Modern World)
Pope John Paul II
The apostolic exhortation issued in 1981on the role of the Christian family

Letter to Families
Pope John Paul II
An encyclical letter to families written during the 1994 Year of the Family.

Mulieris Dignitatum (On the Dignity and Vocation of Women)
Pope John Paul II
This beautiful apostolic letter addresses the issue of the role of women in modern society. Explores the models of women in the Bible and gives a correct understanding of womanhood.

Veritatis Splendor (The Splendor of Truth)
Pope John Paul II
The encyclical letter addresses the fundamental questions of the Church's moral teachings.

Reflections on Humanae Vitae
Pope John Paul II
Addresses of Pope John Paul II to his weekly audiences for six months in 1984, in which he discusses the theology of human love in God's plan.

Donum Vitae (Respect for Human Life)
Congregation for the Doctrine of the Faith
The Church's official position regarding the morality of the various methods of artificial reproduction.

Educational Guidance in Human Love
Sacred Congregation for Catholic Education
The 1983 outlines for Sex Education.

The Truth and Meaning of Human Sexuality
Pontifical Council for the Family
The 1995 Guidelines for Education within the Family.

NFP METHODS, PRACTICAL AND MEDICAL ASPECTS

The Art of Natural Family Planning
John and Sheila Kippley
Comprehensive explanation of the Sympto-thermal Method of the CCL, including the practical, medical, and moral aspects of NFP.

The Medical Application of Natural Family Planning-A Contemporary Approach to Women's Health Care
Dr Thomas W. Hilgers
The Ovulation Method (Creighton Model), NaProTechnology and its application in a medical setting.

The Scientific Foundations of the Ovulation Method
Dr Thomas W. Hilgers
Scientific basis of the Ovulation Method explained.

The Billings Method
Dr Evelyn L. Billings & Ann Westmore
Explanation of the Billings Ovulation Method.

Teaching the Billings Ovulation Method
Drs Evelyn L. & John J. Billings
The two parts volume teaching manual of the Billings Method

THEOLOGICAL AND PHILOSOPHICAL WORKS

Love and Responsibility
Karol Wojtyla
Written before he became Pope John Paul II, this book is an explanation of Catholic vision regarding family life and human sexuality.

Natural Family Planning-Why it Succeeds
Herbert F. Smith, S.J.
Explain the benefits of NFP in a question and answer format.

Catholic Sexual Ethics
Ronald Lawler, Joseph Boyle, Jr, and William May
A summary, explanation and defense of the teachings of the Catholic Church written in complete fidelity to magisterial teachings.

The Teaching of Humanae Vitae—A defense
John C. Ford, SJ, Germain Grisez, Joseph Boyle, John Finnis, and William E. May
Explain why NFP is different from contraception and why this teaching of the Church is binding on all Catholics.

Humanae Vitae: A Generation Later
Janet Smith
Offer a comprehensive, well-written and well-researched text examining the effect and importance of *Humanae Vitae.*

Why Humanae Vitae Was Right: A Reader
Edited by Janet Smith
A collection of some of the best writings on *Humanae Vitae,* including some difficult to locate or out of prints articles. A standard resource on the encyclical.

Marriage and the Family in the Documents of the Magisterium: A Course in the Theology of Marriage
Ramón García de Haro
A work of the late professor of the Pontifical Institute of John Paul II for Studies on Marriage and Family.

A Moral Evaluation of Contraception and Sterilization: A Dialogical Study
Albert Moraczewski and Gary Atkinson
The Pope John XXIII Medical-Moral Research and Education Center publish this work in 1979.

The Bible and Birth Control
Charles D. Provan
Biblical arguments on why contraception is wrong.

Intimate Bedfellows: Love, Sex, and the Catholic Church
Thomas and Donna Finn
A couple reflects on their own journey towards an appreciation of the Church's teaching on marriage and human sexuality. Treat the subjects on pre-marital sex, cohabitation, contraception and responsible parenting.

Sex and the Marriage Covenant
John F. Kippley
Examine the subject of sexuality is systematically examined using the criterion that Sacred Scripture shows that God intends sexual intercourse should be, at least implicitly, a renewal of the marriage covenant.

Birth Control and Christian Discipleship
John F. Kippley
Trace the history of the rejection of contraception in the Protestant traditions, focus on the relationship between contraception and abortion, and more.

In My Mother's Womb
Donald De Marco
Give excellent arguments and explanations of the Catholics Church's defense of human life.

Incarnation in a Divided World
Donald De Marco
An enlightening treatment of the implication of the dogma of Incarnation in areas of human life and ethics.

Margaret Sanger — The Father of American Society
Elasah Drogin
Describe the origin of the birth control movement and the philosophy of Planned Parenthood.

Open Embrace
Sam & Bethany Torode
This couple explains the Scriptural reasons for using NFP from a Protestant perspective.

APPENDIX 4

Of Human Life — A pastoral letter to the people of God of northern Colorado on the truth and meaning of married love

† Charles J. Chaput, O.F.M. Cap. Archbishop of Denver
July 22, 1998

Dear brothers and sisters in the Lord,

1. Thirty years ago this week, Pope Paul VI issued his encyclical letter *Humanae Vitae* (Of Human Life), which reaffirmed the Church's constant teaching on the regulation of births. It is certainly the most misunderstood papal intervention of this century. It was the spark which led to three decades of doubt and dissent among many Catholics, especially in the developed countries. With the passage of time, however, it has also proven prophetic. It teaches the truth. My purpose in this pastoral letter, therefore, is simple. I believe the message of *Humanae Vitae* is not a burden but a joy. I believe this encyclical offers a key to deeper, richer marriages. And so what I seek from the family of our local Church is not just a respectful nod toward a document which critics dismiss as irrelevant, but an active and sustained effort to study *Humanae Vitae*; to teach it faithfully in our parishes; and to encourage our married couples to live it.

I. THE WORLD SINCE 1968

2. Sooner or later, every pastor counsels someone struggling with an addiction. Usually the problem is alcohol or drugs. And usually the scenario is the same. The addict will acknowledge the problem but claim to be powerless against it. Or, alternately, the addict will deny having any problem at all, even if the addiction is destroying his or her health and wrecking job and family. No matter how much sense the pastor makes; no matter how true and persuasive his arguments; and no matter how life-threatening the situation, the addict simply cannot understand — or cannot act on — the counsel. The addiction, like a thick pane of glass, divides the addict from anything or anyone that might help.

3. One way to understand the history of *Humanae Vitae* is to examine the past three decades through this metaphor of addiction. I believe people in the developed world find this encyclical so hard to accept not because of any defect in Paul VI's reasoning, but because of the addictions and contradictions they have inflicted upon themselves, exactly as the Holy Father warned.

4. In presenting his encyclical, Paul VI cautioned against four main problems (HV 17) that would arise if Church teaching on the regulation of births was ignored. First, he warned that the widespread use of contraception would lead to "conjugal infidelity and the general lowering of morality." Exactly this has happened. Few would deny that the rates of abortion, divorce, family breakdown, wife and child abuse, venereal disease and out of wedlock births have all massively increased since the mid-1960s. Obviously, the birth control pill has not been the only factor in this unraveling. But it has played a major role. In fact, the cultural revolution since 1968, driven at least in part by transformed attitudes toward sex, would not have been possible or sustainable without easy access to reliable contraception. In this, Paul VI was right.

5. Second, he also warned that man would lose respect for woman and "no longer [care] for her physical and psychological equilibrium," to the point that he would consider her "as a mere instrument of selfish enjoyment, and no longer as his respected and beloved companion." In other words, according to the Pope, contraception might be marketed as liberating for women, but the real "beneficiaries" of birth control pills and devices would be men. Three decades later, exactly as Paul VI suggested, contraception has released males — to a historically unprecedented degree — from responsibility for their sexual aggression. In the process, one of the stranger ironies of the contraception debate of the past generation has been this: Many feminists have attacked the Catholic Church for her alleged disregard of women, but the Church in *Humanae Vitae* identified and rejected sexual exploitation of women years before that message entered the cultural mainstream. Again, Paul VI was right.

6. Third, the Holy Father also warned that widespread use of contraception would place a "dangerous weapon... in the hands of those public authorities who take no heed of moral exigencies." As we have

since discovered, eugenics didn't disappear with Nazi racial theories in 1945. Population control policies are now an accepted part of nearly every foreign aid discussion. The massive export of contraceptives, abortion and sterilization by the developed world to developing countries — frequently as a prerequisite for aid dollars and often in direct contradiction to local moral traditions — is a thinly disguised form of population warfare and cultural re-engineering. Again, Paul VI was right.

7. Fourth, Pope Paul warned that contraception would mislead human beings into thinking they had unlimited dominion over their own bodies, relentlessly turning the human person into the object of his or her own intrusive power. Herein lies another irony: In fleeing into the false freedom provided by contraception and abortion, an exaggerated feminism has actively colluded in women's dehumanization. A man and a woman participate uniquely in the glory of God by their ability to co-create new life with Him. At the heart of contraception, however, is the assumption that fertility is an infection which must be attacked and controlled, exactly as antibiotics attack bacteria. In this attitude, one can also see the organic link between contraception and abortion. If fertility can be misrepresented as an infection to be attacked, so too can new life. In either case, a defining element of woman's identity — her potential for bearing new life — is recast as a weakness requiring vigilant distrust and "treatment." Woman becomes the object of the tools she relies on to ensure her own liberation and defense, while man takes no share of the burden. Once again, Paul VI was right.

8. From the Holy Father's final point, much more has flowed: *In vitro* fertilization, cloning, genetic manipulation and embryo experimentation are all descendants of contraceptive technology. In fact, we have drastically and naively underestimated the effects of technology not only on external society, but on our own interior human identity. As author Neil Postman has observed, technological change is not additive but ecological. A significant new technology does not "add" something to a society; it changes everything — just as a drop of red dye does not remain discrete in a glass of water, but colors and changes every single molecule of the liquid. Contraceptive technology, precisely because of its impact on sexual intimacy, has subverted our understanding of the purpose of sexuality, fertility and marriage

itself. It has detached them from the natural, organic identity of the human person and disrupted the ecology of human relationships. It has scrambled our vocabulary of love, just as pride scrambled the vocabulary of Babel.

9. Now we deal daily with the consequences. I am writing these thoughts during a July week when, within days of each other, news media have informed us that nearly 14 percent of Coloradans are or have been involved in drug or alcohol dependency; a governor's commission has praised marriage while simultaneously recommending steps that would subvert it in Colorado by extending parallel rights and responsibilities to persons in "committed relationships," including same-sex relationships; and a young east coast couple have been sentenced for brutally slaying their newborn baby. According to news reports, one or both of the young unmarried parents "bashed in [the baby's] skull while he was still alive, and then left his battered body in a Dumpster to die." These are the headlines of a culture in serious distress. U.S. society is wracked with sexual identity and behavior dysfunctions, family collapse and a general coarsening of attitudes toward the sanctity of human life. It's obvious to everyone but an addict: We have a problem. It's killing us as a people. So what are we going to do about it? What I want to suggest is that if Paul VI was right about so many of the consequences deriving from contraception, it is because he was right about contraception itself. In seeking to become whole again as persons and as a people of faith, we need to begin by revisiting *Humanae Vitae* with open hearts. Jesus said the truth would make us free. *Humanae Vitae* is filled with truth. It is therefore a key to our freedom.

II. WHAT HUMANAE VITAE REALLY SAYS

10. Perhaps one of the flaws in communicating the message of Humanae Vitae over the last 30 years has been the language used in teaching it. The duties and responsibilities of married life are numerous. They're also serious. They need to be considered carefully, and prayerfully, in advance. But few couples understand their love in terms of academic theology. Rather, they fall in love. That's the vocabulary they use. It's that simple and revealing. They surrender to each other. They give themselves to each other. They fall into each other in

order to fully possess, and be possessed by, each other. And rightly so. In married love, God intends that spouses should find joy and delight, hope and abundant life, in and through each other — all ordered in a way which draws husband and wife, their children, and all who know them, deeper into God's embrace.

11. As a result, in presenting the nature of Christian marriage to a new generation, we need to articulate its fulfilling satisfactions at least as well as its duties. The Catholic attitude toward sexuality is anything but puritanical, repressive or anti-carnal. God created the world and fashioned the human person in His own image. Therefore the body is good. In fact, it's often been a source of great humor for me to listen incognito as people simultaneously complain about the alleged "bottled-up sexuality" of Catholic moral doctrine, and the size of many good Catholic families. (From where, one might ask, do they think the babies come?) Catholic marriage — exactly like Jesus Himself — is not about scarcity but abundance. It's not about sterility, but rather the fruitfulness which flows from unitive, procreative love. Catholic married love always implies the possibility of new life; and because it does, it drives out loneliness and affirms the future. And because it affirms the future, it becomes a furnace of hope in a world prone to despair. In effect, Catholic marriage is attractive because it is true. It's designed for the creatures we are: persons meant for communion. Spouses complete each other. When God joins a woman and man together in marriage, they create with Him a new wholeness; a "belonging" which is so real, so concrete, that a new life, a child, is its natural expression and seal. This is what the Church means when she teaches that Catholic married love is by its nature both unitive and procreative — not either/or.

12. But why can't a married couple simply choose the unitive aspect of marriage and temporarily block or even permanently prevent its procreative nature? The answer is as simple and radical as the Gospel itself. When spouses give themselves honestly and entirely to each other, as the nature of married love implies and even demands, that must include their whole selves — and the most intimate, powerful part of each person is his or her fertility. Contraception not only denies this fertility and attacks procreation; in doing so, it necessarily damages unity as well. It is the equivalent of spouses saying: "I'll give you all I am — except my fertility; I'll accept all you are — except your

fertility." This withholding of self inevitably works to isolate and divide the spouses, and unravel the holy friendship between them... Maybe not immediately and overtly, but deeply, and in the long run often fatally for the marriage.

13. This is why the Church is not against "artificial" contraception. She is against all contraception. The notion of "artificial" has nothing to do with the issue. In fact, it tends to confuse discussion by implying that the debate is about a mechanical intrusion into the body's organic system. It is not. The Church has no problem with science appropriately intervening to heal or enhance bodily health. Rather, the Church teaches that all contraception is morally wrong; and not only wrong, but seriously wrong. The covenant which husband and wife enter at marriage requires that all intercourse remain open to the transmission of new life. This is what becoming "one flesh" implies: complete self-giving, without reservation or exception, just as Christ withheld nothing of Himself from His bride, the Church, by dying for her on the cross. Any intentional interference with the procreative nature of intercourse necessarily involves spouses' withholding themselves from each other and from God, who is their partner in sacramental love. In effect, they steal something infinitely precious — themselves — from each other and from their Creator.

14. And this is why natural family planning (NFP) differs not merely in style but in moral substance from contraception as a means of regulating family size. NFP is not contraception. Rather, it is a method of fertility awareness and appreciation. It is an entirely different approach to regulating birth. NFP does nothing to attack fertility, withhold the gift of oneself from one's spouse, or block the procreative nature of intercourse. The marriage covenant requires that each act of intercourse be fully an act of self-giving, and therefore open to the possibility of new life. But when, for good reasons, a husband and wife limit their intercourse to the wife's natural periods of infertility during a month, they are simply observing a cycle which God Himself created in the woman. They are not subverting it. And so they are living within the law of God's love.

15. There are, of course, many wonderful benefits to the practice of NFP. The wife preserves herself from intrusive chemicals or devices and remains true to her natural cycle. The husband shares in the plan-

ning and responsibility for NFP. Both learn a greater degree of self-mastery and a deeper respect for each other. It's true that NFP involves sacrifices and periodic abstinence from intercourse. It can, at times, be a difficult road. But so can any serious Christian life, whether ordained, consecrated, single or married. Moreover, the experience of tens of thousands of couples has shown that, when lived prayerfully and unselfishly, NFP deepens and enriches marriage and results in greater intimacy — and greater joy. In the Old Testament, God told our first parents to be fruitful and multiply (Gn 1:28). He told us to choose life (Dt 30:19). He sent His son, Jesus, to bring us life abundantly (Jn 10:10) and to remind us that His yoke is light (Mt 11:30). I suspect, therefore, that at the heart of Catholic ambivalence toward *Humanae Vitae* is not a crisis of sexuality, Church authority or moral relevance, but rather a question of faith: Do we really believe in God's goodness? The Church speaks for her Bridegroom, Jesus Christ, and believers naturally, eagerly listen. She shows married couples the path to enduring love and a culture of life. Thirty years of history record the consequences of choosing otherwise.

III. WHAT WE NEED TO DO

16. I want to express my gratitude to the many couples who already live the message of *Humanae Vitae* in their married lives. Their fidelity to the truth sanctifies their own families and our entire community of faith. I thank in a special way those couples who teach NFP and counsel others in responsible parenthood inspired by Church teaching. Their work too often goes unnoticed or underappreciated-but they are powerful advocates for life in an age of confusion. I also want to offer my prayers and encouragement to those couples who bear the cross of infertility. In a society often bent on avoiding children, they carry the burden of yearning for children but having none. No prayers go unanswered, and all suffering given over to the Lord bears fruit in some form of new life. I encourage them to consider adoption, and I appeal to them to remember that a good end can never justify a wrong means. Whether to prevent a pregnancy or achieve one, all techniques which separate the unitive and procreative dimensions of marriage are always wrong. Procreative techniques which turn embryos into objects and mechanically substitute for the loving embrace of husband and wife violate human dignity and treat life as a product. No matter

how positive their intentions, these techniques advance the dangerous tendency to reduce human life to material which can be manipulated.

17. It's never too late to turn our hearts back toward God. We are not powerless. We can make a difference by witnessing the truth about married love and fidelity to the culture around us. In December last year, in a pastoral letter entitled Good News of Great Joy, I spoke of the important vocation every Catholic has as an evangelizer. We are all missionaries. America in the 1990s, with its culture of disordered sexuality, broken marriages and fragmented families, urgently needs the Gospel. As Pope John Paul II writes in his apostolic exhortation On the Family *(Familiaris Consortio)*, married couples and families have a critical role in witnessing Jesus Christ to each other and to the surrounding culture (49, 50).

18. In that light, I ask married couples of the archdiocese to read, discuss and pray over *Humanae Vitae, Familiaris Consortio* and other documents of the Church which outline Catholic teaching on marriage and sexuality. Many married couples, unaware of the valuable wisdom found in these materials, have deprived themselves of a beautiful source of support for their mutual love. I especially encourage couples to examine their own consciences regarding contraception, and I ask them to remember that "conscience" is much more than a matter of personal preference. It requires us to search out and understand Church teaching, and to honestly strive to conform our hearts to it. I urge them to seek sacramental Reconciliation for the times they may have fallen into contraception. Disordered sexuality is the dominant addiction of American society in these closing years of the century. It directly or indirectly impacts us all. As a result, for many, this teaching may be a hard message to accept. But do not lose heart. Each of us is a sinner. Each of us is loved by God. No matter how often we fail, God will deliver us if we repent and ask for the grace to do His will.

19. I ask my brother priests to examine their own pastoral practices, to ensure that they faithfully and persuasively present the Church's teaching on these issues in all their parish work. Our people deserve the truth about human sexuality and the dignity of marriage. To accomplish this, I ask pastors to read and implement the Vademecum for Confessors Concerning Some Aspects of the Morality of Conjugal Life, and to study the Church's teaching on marriage and family planning. I urge them to

appoint parish coordinators to facilitate the presentation of Catholic teaching on married love and family planning — especially NFP. Contraception is a grave matter. Married couples need the good counsel of the Church to make right decisions. Most married Catholics welcome the guidance of their priests, and priests should never feel intimidated by their personal commitment to celibacy, or embarrassed by the teaching of the Church. To be embarrassed by Church teaching is to be embarrassed by Christ's teaching. The pastoral experience and counsel of a priest are valuable on issues like contraception precisely because he brings new perspective to a couple and speaks for the whole Church. Moreover, the fidelity a priest shows to his own vocation strengthens married people to live their vocation more faithfully.

20. As archbishop, I commit myself and my offices to supporting my brother priests, deacons and their lay collaborators in presenting the whole of the Church's teaching on married love and family planning. I owe both the clergy of our local Church and their staffs — especially the many dedicated parish catechists — much gratitude for the good work they have already accomplished in this area. It is my intention to ensure that courses on married love and family planning are available on a regular basis to more and more people of the archdiocese, and that our priests and deacons receive more extensive education in the theological and pastoral aspects of these issues. I direct, in a particular way, our Offices of Evangelization and Catechetics; Marriage and Family Life; Catholic Schools; Youth, Young Adult and Campus Ministries; and the Rite of Christian Initiation for Adults to develop concrete ways to better present Church teaching on married love to our people, and to require adequate instruction in NFP as part of all marriage preparation programs in the archdiocese.

21. Two final points. First, the issue of contraception is not peripheral, but central and serious in a Catholic's walk with God. If knowingly and freely engaged in, contraception is a grave sin, because it distorts the essence of marriage: the self-giving love which, by its very nature, is life-giving. It breaks apart what God created to be whole: the person-uniting meaning of sex (love) and the life-giving meaning of sex (procreation). Quite apart from its cost to individual marriages, contraception has also inflicted massive damage on society at large: initially by driving a wedge between love and the procreation of children; and then between sex (i.e., Recreational sex without permanent commitment) and love.

Nonetheless — and this is my second point — teaching the truth should always be done with patience and compassion, as well as firmness. American society seems to swing peculiarly between puritanism and license. The two generations — my own and my teachers' — which once led the dissent from Paul VI's encyclical in this country, are generations still reacting against the American Catholic rigorism of the 1950s. That rigorism, much of it a product of culture and not doctrine, has long since been demolished. But the habit of skepticism remains. In reaching these people, our task is to turn their distrust to where it belongs: toward the lies the world tells about the meaning of human sexuality, and the pathologies those lies conceal.

22. In closing, we face an opportunity which comes only once in many decades. Thirty years ago this week, Paul VI told the truth about married love. In doing it, he triggered a struggle within the Church which continues to mark American Catholic life even today. Selective dissent from *Humanae Vitae* soon fueled broad dissent from Church authority and attacks on the credibility of the Church herself. The irony is that the people who dismissed Church teaching in the 1960s soon discovered that they had subverted their own ability to pass anything along to their children. The result is that the Church now must evangelize a world of their children's children — adolescents and young adults raised in moral confusion, often unaware of their own moral heritage, who hunger for meaning, community, and love with real substance. For all its challenges, this is a tremendous new moment of possibility for the Church, and the good news is that the Church today, as in every age, has the answers to fill the God-shaped empty places in their hearts. My prayer is therefore simple: May the Lord grant us the wisdom to recognize the great treasure which resides in our teaching about married love and human sexuality, the faith, joy and perseverance to live it in our own families — and the courage which Paul VI possessed to preach it anew.

† Charles J. Chaput, O.F.M. Cap. Archbishop of Denver, July 22, 1998.

ADDENDUM: SOME COMMON QUESTIONS

In the weeks following publication of his pastoral letter, Archbishop Chaput answered some common questions about family planning and related issues in his regular Denver Catholic Register column.

1. Isn't a couple's method of family planning a matter of personal conscience?

Yes it is. Catholics, like all people, are always obligated to follow their consciences — on birth control and every other matter. But that's not where the problem lies. The problem lies in the formation of one's conscience. A conscientious person seeks to do good and avoid evil. Seeing the difference between good and evil, though, can sometimes be difficult. As Pope John Paul II has said, the basic moral law is written in the human heart because we're created in the image and likeness of God. But we bear the wounds of original sin, which garbles the message and dims our ability to judge and act according to truth.

Truth is objective. In other words, it's real; independent of us; and exists whether we like it or not. Therefore, conscience can't invent right and wrong. Rather, conscience is called to discover the truth of right and wrong, and then to submit personal judgments to the truth once it is found. Church teaching on the regulation of births, like all her moral teachings, is a sure guide for forming our consciences according to the truth. For we have the certainty of faith, as Vatican II reminds us, that the teachings of the Church on matters of faith and morals are "not the mere word of men, but truly the word of God" (*Lumen Gentium* n. 12). Too often, we use "conscience" as a synonym for private preference; a kind of pious alibi for doing what we want or taking the easy road. We only end up hurting others and ourselves.

2. I still don't see the big difference between a couple using "artificial" birth control and a couple using "natural" family planning. Don't both couples have the same intention, and isn't this what determines morality?

It's hard to see the difference when the emphasis is placed on "artificial" versus "natural" methods. People rightly point out that many things we use are artificial but not immoral. So it's important to realize that the Church doesn't oppose artificial birth control because it's artificial.

Rather, what the Church opposes is any method of birth control which is contraceptive, whether artificial devices, pills, etc., Are used or not. Contraception is the choice, by any means, to sterilize a given act of intercourse. In other words, a contracepting couple chooses to engage in intercourse and, knowing that it may result in a new life, they intentionally and willfully suppress their fertility. Herein lies a key distinction: Natural family planning (NFP) is in no way contraceptive. The choice to abstain from a fertile act of intercourse is completely different from the willful choice to sterilize a fertile act of intercourse. NFP simply accepts from God's hand the natural cycle of infertility that He has built into the nature of woman.

Regarding the issue of intention: Yes, both couples may have the same end in mind — to avoid pregnancy. But the means to achieve their common goal are not at all alike. Take, for example, two students, each of whom intends to excel in school. Obviously that's a very good intention. With the same goal in mind, one studies diligently. The other cheats on every test. The point is, the end doesn't justify the means — in getting an education, in regulating births, or in anything else.

3. *I'm a priest. If I preach about what's wrong with contraception, I'll lose people.*

Let me turn that around: If priests don't preach the Church's message about contraception, heaven loses people. Don't be afraid. When Jesus preached the truth, He lost people. But, little by little, He gained even more people. Take courage in the Lord.

It shouldn't surprise us that people find this teaching hard to accept. Every Gospel-based life has things which are hard to accept. Should we stop teaching the truth because it's difficult? Of course not. We have the joy and the responsibility before God to preach the truth lovingly in season and out of season. The Church won't be renewed without a renewal of family life. And the family can't be renewed without a return to the truths taught in *Humanae Vitae.* Ignoring this issue can't be an option: In the long run, its cost is too high. Therefore, we should make every effort to better understand the importance of Church teaching in this regard, and witness to it boldly and with confidence.

4. *In your pastoral letter, you said that the most intimate, powerful part of each person is his or her fertility. My husband and I are unable to have children. What does this mean for us?*

Many couples bear a great cross because, despite their openness to life, they're unable to have children. But marital love is always life-giving when spouses give themselves honestly to each other, even if a child isn't conceived. Only when husband and wife intentionally withhold their fertility, or abuse their sexuality in some other way, can we speak of a "life-less" act of intercourse.

Spouses' self-giving in one flesh remains the most intimate, powerful and life-giving expression of their love for one another, even when nature, or some problem of nature, prevents new life from being conceived. Medical technology can sometimes correct a physical problem, allowing a child to be conceived by the loving embrace of parents. This is a proper and wonderful use of technology. However, couples should remember that, as creatures themselves, they're not the arbiters of human life. Ultimately, no one is free to manipulate the conception of a human person. No matter how sincere a couple's intentions, many of today's new procreative techniques treat human life as a product which can be manufactured — and in doing so, they violate human dignity. Again, the end never justifies the means.

Children aren't the only way a marriage can be fruitful. If God, in His design, closes one option for a couple, He will open another. Their love can find expression in adoption, foster-parenting, or dozens of forms of apostolic work. This kind of counsel, of course, is much easier to give than to willingly accept. I would never want to understate the real pain and loss felt by infertile couples. But I know, both from faith and from my friendships with married couples over the years, that if a husband and wife choose to trust God, their love will always be rewarded with fertility and new life — if not in the form of a child, then in the way they impact the world around them.

5. Why is the Church so obsessed with sex?

You know the old saying about the pot calling the kettle black — well, here's a great example. Questions like this one may very well be honest, but they conceal where the real obsessions lie. American society is drowning in a sea of disordered sexuality. In such circumstances, it's hardly an "obsession" for the Church to speak clearly and forcefully about how to swim. It's her responsibility and mission.

God created our sexuality to be a sign in the world of His own life and love, and to reveal to us that we can only fulfill ourselves by loving as He loves. When sexuality becomes distorted, however, it's no longer able to communicate God's life and love. Empty of true love, life lacks meaning, and people soon seem disposable. Sex becomes a pursuit of selfish gratification at the expense of others. Children are no longer welcomed as the natural fruit of married love, but are seen as a burden to be avoided. We don't even shrink from killing (through abortion) thousands of innocent preborn lives a day in satisfying our convenience and appetites.

It's no exaggeration, then, to say that disordered sexuality is the beginning of what Pope John Paul II calls "the culture of death." In fact, we'll never build a culture of life and love without first restoring the true meaning of human sexuality. If the Church is so concerned about sex, it's because she seeks to defend the dignity of the human person, and to safeguard the true meaning of life and love which sexuality is meant to reveal.

6. *How can I preach against contraception and praise the virtues of NFP? As a priest, I'm not married.*

First, the truth is the truth, no matter who speaks it. Second, preaching isn't about the preacher; it's about the message. Third, in his promise of celibacy, a priest doesn't forget or deny his sexuality. Instead, he dedicates it to a different — but equally fertile — kind of fruitfulness. In other words, priestly celibacy is an affirmation, not a rejection; a strength, not a weakness. It's a "yes" to God which enables us to understand and serve our people better.

Remember that marriage, religious life, the single vocation and the priesthood are all designed to fit together and complement each other in the life of the Church. Each needs the other. Each, in its own proper way, fulfills the fundamental human vocation to give ourselves away in love. I think we priests often underestimate how effective our pastoral counsel can be on issues like contraception. People want and need the truth, and over time, the human heart naturally responds to it. But our people can't respond if they don't hear the message of *Humanae Vitae* faithfully and persuasively from their pastors. That's our job, and we should embrace it joyfully.

INDEX